City

nantha Taylor

www.heinemann.co.uk

✓ Free online support
✓ Useful weblinks
✓ 24 hour online ordering

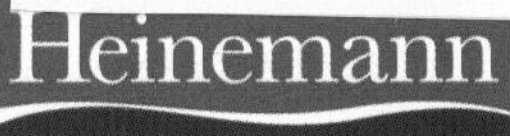

Inspi

Harcourt Education Limited
Halley Court, Jordan Hill, Oxford OX2 8EJ

Heinemann is the registered trademark of
Harcourt Education Limited

First published 2006

11 10 09 08 07 06
10 9 8 7 6 5 4 3 2 1

British Library Cataloguing in Publication Data is available
from the British Library on request.

10-digit ISBN: 0 435 46307 1
13-digit ISBN: 978 0 435 46307 6

Edited by Susan Ross (Ross Economics and Editorial Services Ltd)
Designed by GD Associates
Layout by Bigtop
Printed in the UK by Bath Colour
Illustrated by Darren Lingard and Luke Walwyn

Cover design by Wooden Ark
Cover photo: © Corbis
Picture research by Ruth Blair

Websites

Please note that the examples of websites suggested in this book were up to date at the time of writing. We have made all links available on the Heinemann website at www.heinemann.co.uk/hotlinks. When you access the site, the express code is 3071P.

Contents

Acknowledgements

Gilly Ford would like to thank: my family for all their support, especially my mum for teaching me to believe in myself. To all my friends that helped on the photo shoot (Andrea Long, Danielle Long, Kathryn Shaw, Kirsty Preston and Kris Arkwright), I am extremely grateful for your contribution.

Helen Stewart would like to thank: Ade, Paul and Mike for all their love and support.

Thanks to all the models who took part in the photo shoot: Kris Arkwright, Samantha Higgins, Cherie Lewis, Vicky Lester, Andrea Long, Danielle Long, Kirsty Preston, Attiqur Rehman, Kathryn Shaw and Victoria Smalley. You were so wonderful, patient and professional, even though you had to sit around for long periods of time! Thanks also to South Trafford College for the use of their facilities during the shoot.

Many thanks to James Bremner at Shortcuts Software UK for supplying photos.

The i-salon computer system screen graphic on p40 courtesy of Integrity Software.

A huge thank you to Glen Burr for providing the hair stylist job profile on p176 and the amazing photos on p86, 110, 123 and 177.

Many thanks to Alex Bickers at TIGI for all her help with the product images on p100. For more information on TIGI products visit www.tigi.co.uk.

Thanks to Philippa Jenkins at L'Oréal for the product image on p100.

Thanks to Reed Business Information for permission to reproduce the Hairdressers Journal International cover on p185.

Photos

ADF Management, p132; Alamy, p179; Art Directors, p84; Jordan Burr Associates, p86, p110, p123, p177 (top); Corbis, p52; Getty Images, p34 (top); Getty Images/PhotoDisc, p139; Harcourt Education/Gareth Boden, p11, p34 (bottom), p35 (top), p46, p60 (top), p61 (right), p69, p93, p101 (round brushes, vent brush, dressing out brush), p102 (hood dryer, neck brush, back mirror, neat section), p114 (rods, combs), p115 (bowl, combs, brush), p116 (gown), p118, p126, p154, p162 (spatula), p163–164, p166, p171, p176, p177 (bottom); Harcourt Education/Chris Honeywell, p61 (left), p95, p97, p100 (bottom), p102 (diffuser), p105 (rollers), p114 (papers), p116 (towels, cotton wool), p121–122; Harcourt Education/Peter Morris, p144, p162 (file, stick); Daniel Lee, p14; Lindos, p35 (bottom); Mack Hairdressing, Chelmsford, p26; PhotoDisc, p51 (bottom); Science Photo Library, p92, p98, p140, p141; Scissors, p28; Wella, p101 (hand dryer and nozzle attachment); www.photos.com, p82.

Special thanks to Julia Conway for permission to reproduce photos on pages 138, 174 and 181.

Product images on page 100 courtesy of L'ORÉAL PROFESSIONNEL and TIGI.

All other photos copyright Harcourt Education/Jules Selmes.

Every effort has been made to contact copyright holders of material reproduced in this book. Any omissions will be rectified in subsequent impressions if notice is given to the publishers.

Introduction

This book has been written to help you achieve your City & Guilds Level 1 Certificate in Salon Services. It has been designed to provide you with all the information you need to guide you through the qualification, with lots of technical information and advice from the experts, including step by step photographs and illustrations of hairdressing and beauty therapy tasks.

Some of the units are just about hairdressing, some are just about beauty therapy, and some units relate to both (known as generic units).

Generic units

1 Customer service

2 Salon reception

3 Personal presentation

4 Health and safety

9 Working in hair and beauty

Hairdressing units

5 Hairdressing services

6 Perming and colouring

Beauty therapy units

7 Basic make-up

8 Basic manicure

About City & Guilds Level 1 Certificate in Salon Services

This qualification is for anyone at any age (but in particular young learners at Key Stage 4) who wants to follow a career in either hairdressing or beauty therapy. You will have the opportunity to experience your chosen industry whilst developing essential life skills and background knowledge.

The qualification gives a good introduction to working in hair or beauty – you can begin to develop the necessary skills without having to show occupational competence, as is necessary when completing an NVQ qualification.

To achieve the full qualification, **all nine units** must be completed. However, you may chose to follow either a hairdressing or a beauty therapy route, in which case you must complete all **five generic units** plus the **two** subject-specific units. This means if you are doing just hairdressing or just beauty therapy, your qualification will be made up of **seven units** in total.

This qualification aims to provide you with:

- Knowledge and skills that will help you whether you choose to work in hairdressing or beauty therapy, continue in general education or go into another area of vocational learning
- A background understanding of the hairdressing or beauty therapy industry and the skills required to work in them
- Knowledge of the kind of work that is involved in hair and beauty, helping you to decide whether this is the right career for you
- A chance to decide if you have the right personal skills to work in hair or beauty
- A general insight into the world of work

Methods of assessment

While you are working towards this qualification you will be assessed in a number of different ways:

- **Practical assessment** – you will actually carry out a hairdressing or beauty therapy task (e.g. winding a perm or giving a basic manicure)
- **Assignments** – you will carry out simple research tasks that ask you to look at trends and fashions and find out about different parts of the hair and beauty industry. You will add assignments and other information to your portfolio
- **Multiple-choice test** – you will have to answer 40 questions (eight from each of the five generic units). You can use the Check what you know questions at the end of each unit in this book to help you practice

Features of this book

As you read through this book, you will notice several special features:

- Glossary – some of the words used in this book might be new to you, especially if they are technical. They appear in a different colour and the meaning can be found in the margin (like here!)
- Safe! – health and safety information to help you work safely in the salon
- Top Tips – great pieces of advice that will help you work professionally
- Salon scene – a real life situation from a salon with questions that get you to think about what happened and what you might have done in the same situation
- Dear Nat – problems or issues that you may come across in the salon. Nat will always have good advice which will help if you find yourself in a similar situation
- Try it out! – fun activities or tasks that get you to think about or build on what you have read
- Over to you – activities to help you build up your portfolio. You may need to carry out some research and then write a short assignment. Quite often you will need to collect photographs or pictures to illustrate your assignments
- A day in the life of – an idea of what an average day working in a salon might be like (found in Unit 9)
- Check what you know – at the end of each unit you can make sure you have understood and remembered what you have learned so far

words or phrases that need special knowledge to understand

Some extra help

You can download a free useful information sheet by visiting www.heinemann.co.uk (just click the FE & Vocational link, and then the Hair & Beauty tab). The sheet contains the following information:

- Getting the most out of reading – why it is important to read and what type of stuff you should be reading.
- Successful internet research – getting the most out of the internet, including how to use search engines and access the most useful websites.
- Creating your portfolio – getting started, presenting information in the best possible way, plus some useful tips on writing your assignments.
- How to write a short report – useful advice on planning and writing a short report.
- Study and revision skills – the best way to study and revise for success.

You can also access links to useful and interesting websites by visiting www.heinemann.co.uk/hotlinks. Just enter the express code 3071P.

We wish you the best of luck and hope you enjoy finding out more about working in the exciting world of hair and beauty!

Gilly Ford, Helen Stewart and Samantha Taylor

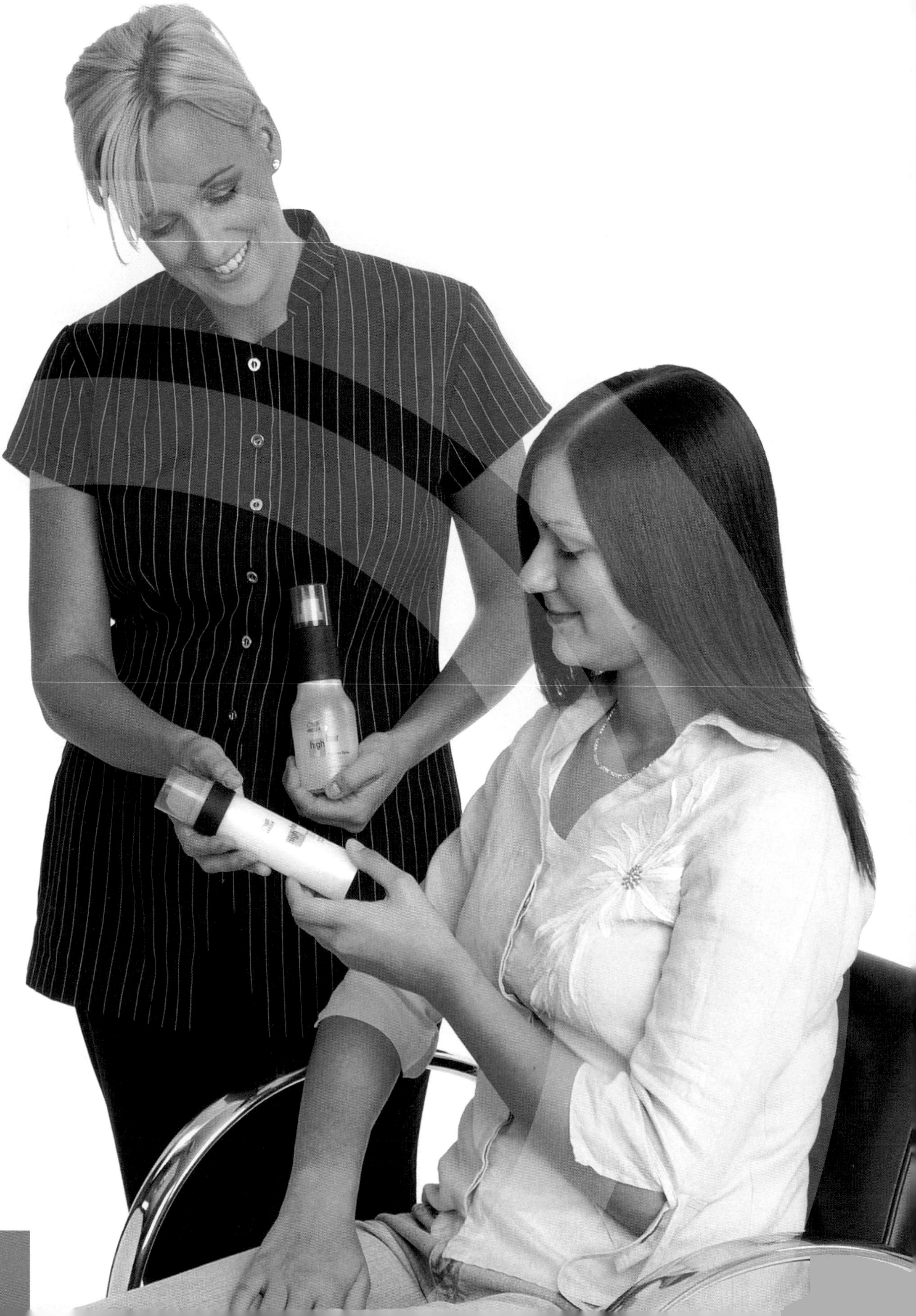

Unit 1

Customer service

Imagine you're a customer going into a salon for the first time. You stand in the reception area and everyone ignores you! How would you feel? Now imagine going into the same salon, but this time you're greeted with a smile and 'Good morning, how can I help you?'. Now how would you feel? Customers are very important people. It is likely that this will be your first experience of dealing with the public, so this unit is all about dealing with customers while working in a salon.

In this unit you will learn about:

- Aspects of customer service.
- Good team working.
- Professional attitudes and behaviour.

Towards the end of this unit, you will be observed and assessed on:

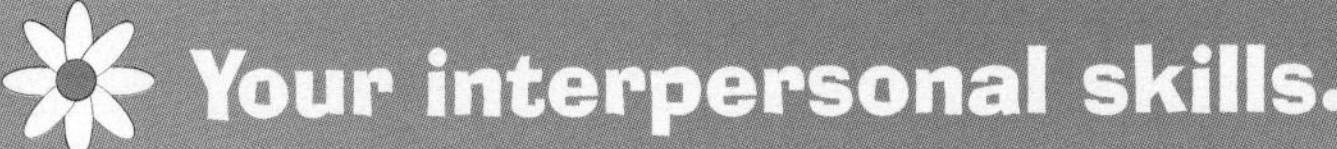

- Your interpersonal skills.

Aspects of customer service

What is customer service?

First, let's look at the meaning of 'customer service'. Who are 'customers' in terms of salon work? They are all the clients you deal with – whether having a blow-dry or a manicure or simply buying a product. Next, think about the word 'service'. This means that you have helped in some way to provide hair or beauty treatments to the salon's clients, however small your role might be, for example taking and hanging up a customer's coat, or making the customer a coffee. Everything you do in the salon offers customer service and that's why it is an important part of your work role!

Communication skills

You communicate in many different ways in everything you do. Think about the four main ways you will communicate with clients in the salon. They are:

- Face-to-face.
- Telephone.
- Written.
- Electronic communication.

No matter which one of these you use, you must always be professional in the way you carry it out.

having high working standards with a good attitude

Face-to-face communication

Face-to-face communication involves using both verbal and non-verbal skills. This means the way you talk and the way you use body language such as smiling, nodding or listening.

TRY IT OUT!

Look at these two illustrations and decide which one looks the most professional and why.

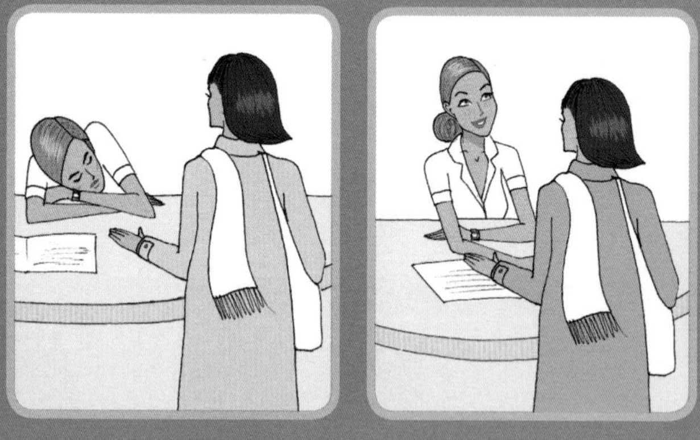

Eye contact shows a client that you are interested in what he or she is saying. If you are unable to give the client your full attention, then excuse yourself politely and deal with whatever is stopping you from concentrating fully on the client. You must remember to return and not get sidetracked!

You will also need to speak clearly – don't put your hands in front of your face or chew gum or sweets. If you are struggling to understand what a client needs, then ask a senior member of staff for help – this also shows your professionalism.

Using the telephone

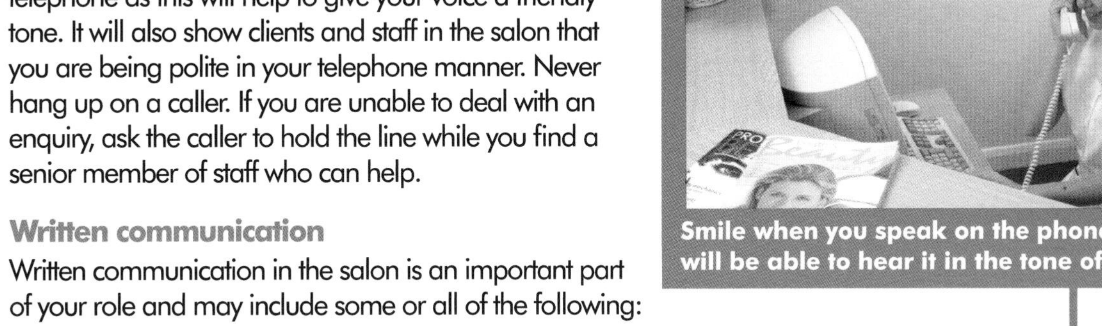

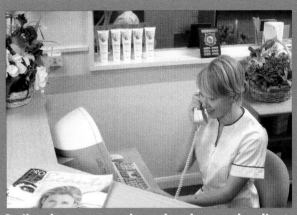

Smile when you speak on the phone – the client will be able to hear it in the tone of your voice

Find out what the correct telephone greeting is for your salon. It will probably be something like 'Good morning/afternoon, Hair Academy, Natalie speaking, how can I help you?' It is important to smile as you speak on the telephone as this will help to give your voice a friendly tone. It will also show clients and staff in the salon that you are being polite in your telephone manner. Never hang up on a caller. If you are unable to deal with an enquiry, ask the caller to hold the line while you find a senior member of staff who can help.

Written communication

Written communication in the salon is an important part of your role and may include some or all of the following:

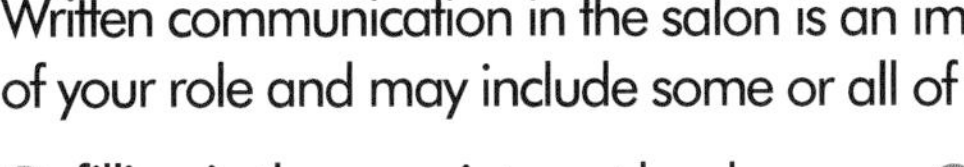

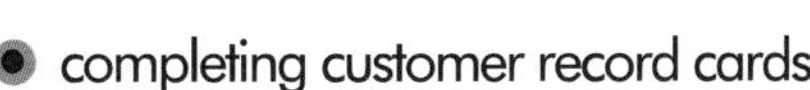

- filling in the appointment book
- taking messages
- completing customer record cards
- completing a stock check list.

The **appointment book** is an essential part of the day-to-day running of the salon. If the appointment system fails, it can throw the whole salon day into chaos! Before you begin to use the appointment book, make sure that you have a good understanding of how it works. Always write neatly – other members of staff must be able to read your writing.

TRY IT OUT!

Write down a list of the abbreviations used in the appointment book. Beside each abbreviation write down what it means and then add the expected time or duration of each service in your salon. Two examples have been done for you.

Abbreviation	Meaning	Service time
B/W	Blow wave	30 minutes
Man/Ped	Manicure and pedicure	30 minutes

Compare your list with others in your group. You will find it interesting to see the variations in the abbreviations used and the timings allowed. Making this list will help you to remember the system used for booking appointments in your salon.

Client record cards are an essential and very important written record of the exact service the client has had. The information written on the card must be accurate to prevent any mistakes being made in future. Remember that record cards may be used as evidence if a client decides to bring a court case against the salon, so every detail must be carefully written down. If you are asked to complete a client record card, always check the client's personal details are correct – they might have changed. Never fill out a card if you are unsure about what to write.

FACIAL TREATMENT | NAME | TEL | HOME | OFFICE | AGE

ADDRESS

DOCTOR Name: | TEL : | SMOKE | DRINK | MEDICATION:

MEDICAL HISTORY | ASTHMA | HEPATITIS | DIABETES | ALLERGIES:

GENERAL HEALTH | GOOD | POOR | CONSTIPATION | BLOOD PRESSURE | NORMAL | HIGH | LOW

SKIN ASSESSMENT	A	B	C		A	B	C		A	B	C
SEBORRHOEA				DELICATE				SUNTAN			
OPEN PORES				DRY				PIGMENTATION			
BLOCKED PORES				DEHYDRATED				DILATED CAPILLARIES			
BLACKHEADS				MATURE				SKINTAGS			
ACNE				AGEING				MOLES			
SCARS				SLACK				SUPERFLUOUS HAIR			

	TREATMENT	MACHINE SETTINGS	PRODUCTS	AMPOULES	ADVISED FOR FOR HOME USE	THERAPIST	AMOUNT £	DATE
1								
2								
3								
4								
5								
6								

HOMECARE ROUTINE: ADVICE FOLLOWED YES ☐ NO ☐ REGULAR HOME USE ☐ IRREGULAR HOME USE ☐

NOTES

INDEMNITY: I confirm that to the best of my knowledge the answers that I have given are correct and that I have not withheld any information that may be relevant to my treatment.

Signature .... Date ....

A client record card

When taking a **message**, make sure you write down the person's name and contact details accurately so that the person the message is for has all the information he or she needs. It is also a good idea to note the date and time the message was taken to prevent any misunderstanding.

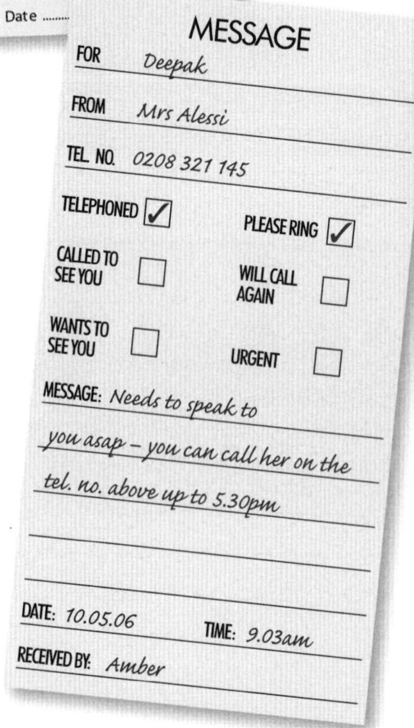

MESSAGE

FOR *Deepak*

FROM *Mrs Alessi*

TEL. NO. *0208 321 145*

TELEPHONED ☑ PLEASE RING ☑

CALLED TO SEE YOU ☐ WILL CALL AGAIN ☐

WANTS TO SEE YOU ☐ URGENT ☐

MESSAGE: *Needs to speak to you asap – you can call her on the tel. no. above up to 5.30pm*

DATE: *10.05.06* TIME: *9.03am*

RECEIVED BY: *Amber*

A message slip

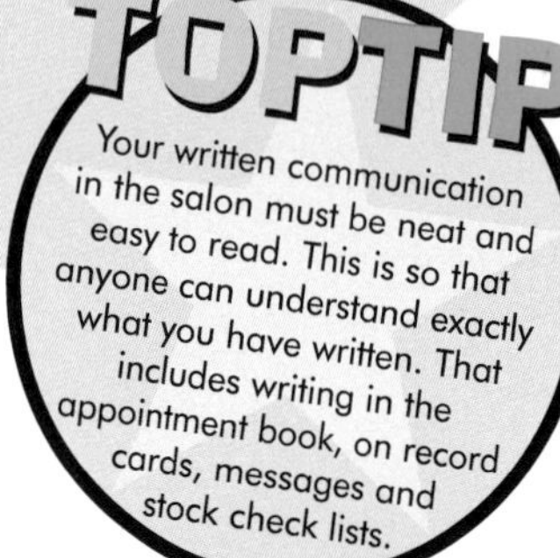

TOPTIP
Your written communication in the salon must be neat and easy to read. This is so that anyone can understand exactly what you have written. That includes writing in the appointment book, on record cards, messages and stock check lists.

You may be asked to take part in a stock check which will involve completing a **stock check list**. You must fill this out fully and accurately to prevent any over or under ordering of stock. Too much or too little stock can cause serious problems in the day-to-day running of the salon.

STOCKINFO

Date: 25/05/03

Description	Product ref	Reorder level	Instock	Quantity required
Control Shampoo 250ml	8385	10	8	10
Control Conditioner 150 ml	8275	10	4	12
Control Shine Serum 50 ml	8573	10	5	8
Control Gel 30 ml	9835	10	6	8
Active Shampoo 250 ml	8935	10	9	12
Active Conditioner 150 ml	9275	10	5	10
Active Shine Serum 50 ml	4625	10	4	7
Active Gel 30 ml	3857	10	7	6
Style Shampoo 250 ml	2746	10	8	12
Style Conditioner 150 ml	6236	10	2	15
Style Shine Serum 50 ml	5254	10	5	6
Style Gel 30 ml	3646	10	3	4

Ordered by: Ros

A stock check list

Electronic communication

If the salon has a computer system, you are likely to be trained in how to use it. This may involve updating client records, recording stock or booking appointments. Use the system only if you fully understand how to do so. Ask for further training if you are unsure. Efficient use of the system will help to ensure the smooth running of the salon.

> If you are using a computer for long periods, make sure you are seated comfortably and take regular breaks to prevent you from feeling tired or developing problems with your posture.

posture: the way you sit or stand

The basics of customer service

Satisfied clients make a successful business! You will need to understand what pleases clients – in terms of their needs, expectations, experience and satisfaction – in order to ensure a healthy business.

Clients' **needs** are the services or products that they require from the salon. Their **expectations** are how they think these should be provided. For example they may expect the salon to be open late evenings, as they work until 5 pm, or that they can pay by credit or debit card rather than in cash. If their expectations are not met, then they will take their business elsewhere.

The clients' **experience** of the salon is the time they spend dealing with the salon, including phone calls to make appointments as well as the time spent having a service. Client **satisfaction** refers to how happy clients are with the service or product provided. Are they pleased enough to return for further services? Will they recommend the salon to others? This is what every salon would like to achieve!

TRY IT OUT!

Think about what makes you feel good when you go into a shop and receive excellent customer service. If the staff are polite, how does that make you feel? If they help you out and thank you for your custom, does that make you feel special? Write a brief account of when you have had a good experience of being a customer. If you can't think of one, ask a family member or friend about their experiences.

Your employer will require you to uphold the image of the salon. This means you must be friendly, helpful, reliable and able to use your own initiative.

initiative: able to complete tasks for yourself without having to be told

You need to keep asking yourself: am I providing clients with a quality service and value for money? The way you perform each task in the salon – in fact your whole attitude – will convince clients that you are giving them the right experience. These are some examples of positive customer experiences:

- Smiling and greeting the client politely as he or she enters the salon.
- Taking the client's coat and offering a seat or refreshments.
- Taking messages accurately at reception.
- Completing a service in the professionally recommended time, so as not to delay the client.
- Completing the appointment book accurately to avoid double booking or disappointing a client.
- Staying calm when dealing with a stressful situation, especially if the client is angry or confused.

All of them will help you to display a **professional attitude**.

Services and products of the salon

When you are shopping, what makes you interested in what a shop has to offer? Value for money? Eye-catching displays of products? Your salon's clients will probably feel the same way about your salon. It may even be your job to keep the product displays clean, tidy and well stocked.

The services and products offered by your salon are the foundations of the business. Without them there would be no salon, and that is why it is important for you to have good service and product knowledge. You will need a basic knowledge of all the services your salon offers, their prices and how long they take. You should also be aware of the product ranges that the salon offers and the prices on the price list. Thorough service and product knowledge will impress both the clients and your boss!

foundations: the base on which something stands

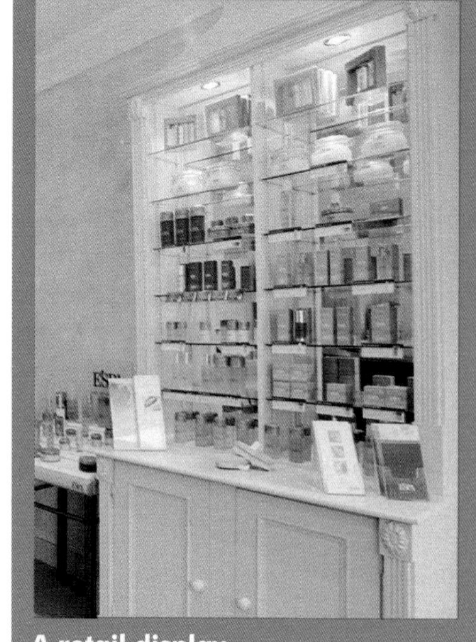

A retail display

If a client asks a question about a product or service and you do not know the answer, always ask a senior member of staff for more information. There are laws against giving customers false or misleading information – you'll need to remember this every time you deal with a query from a client.

TRY IT OUT!

Write a list of products and services offered in the salon where you work. Beside each product/service, note down its price and in the case of a service, the time it takes to do. Being familiar with this type of information will also help you in the work you do at reception.

Differing customer needs and expectations

What does differing customer needs and expectations mean? It means that no two people want the same service or expect the same treatment. This means you have a big task on your hands to please everyone all of the time! That would be easy if we lived in a perfect world, but no one can be perfect all of the time. Instead, you can work hard to provide an excellent all-round salon service to all of the clients that come into the salon. This will involve adapting the way you speak to and deal with each client. For example, you would talk differently to a client of your own age than to an elderly client.

All clients need different things and this will affect how your salon is run. For example, if your salon is in a busy city centre, then you will need to cater for busy, young clients and have a fresh and modern approach. If your salon is in a residential area, you are likely to have a mix of clients such as young families and older people. The salon you work for also has a responsibility to provide services that people with disabilities can use, for example a ramp outside the salon.

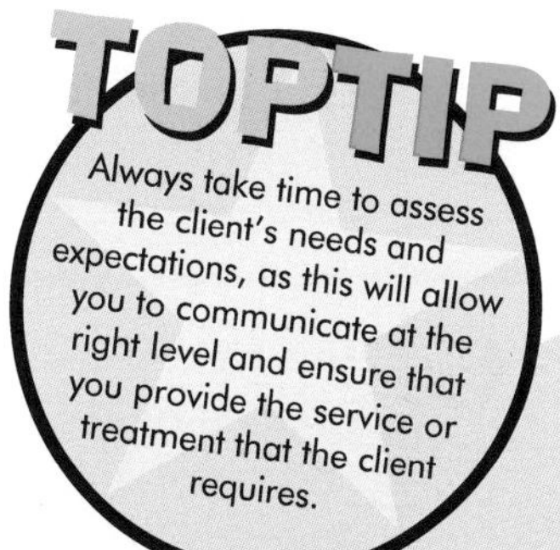

TOPTIP
Always take time to assess the client's needs and expectations, as this will allow you to communicate at the right level and ensure that you provide the service or treatment that the client requires.

OVER TO YOU...

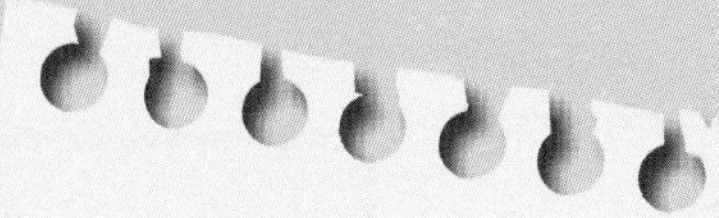

Visit a range of salons in your area to see what sort of image each has, e.g. fashionable, no-frills, expensive/inexpensive. Look at salon names – do they reflect the image that the salon is trying to present? Write a short report describing different salon images. If you wish, you can include sketches, pictures from magazines or photographs.

Good team working

Personality types

Your personality is all about the way you act and communicate with other people. The three personality types you need to be aware of and that may affect your working life are:

- Passive.
- Assertive.
- Aggressive.

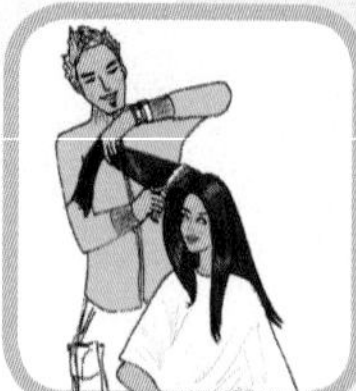
Passive personality

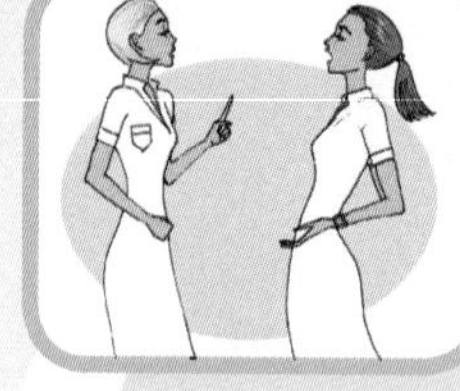
Assertive personality

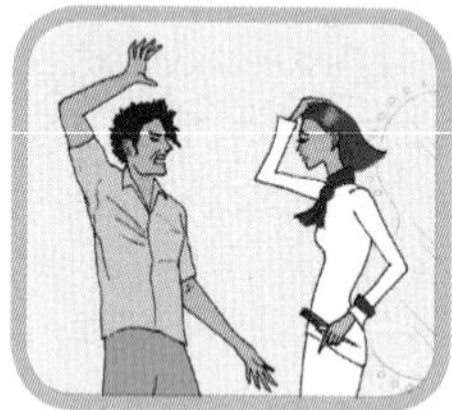
Aggressive personality

Of course, your personality can be described in other ways, but if you know about the three above and how to handle these types of personality in both clients and other staff members, it will help your working relations in the salon. You may find yourself described in the table below!

Personality types

Personality	Client	Staff
Passive	This type of client is patient and easily pleased. He or she is relaxed in their outlook and on life in general, and rarely causes a fuss.	This type of staff member is usually easy to get along with but may lack enthusiam for his or her work which can cause problems. He or she is happy to sit back and let others put in all the effort.
Assertive	This type of client knows what he or she wants and is not afraid to be honest with you. This will only cause problems if you are the sort of person who finds it hard to take criticism.	This type of staff member will not be bossed around and will challenge anything that he or she feels is unfair. However, assertive people will often try to take over and succeed in having things their way, especially if other staff members are passive.
Aggressive	This type of client can be very difficult to work with, often being unnecessarily critical and offensive. Always try to remain calm and polite when dealing with aggressive clients.	Staff members that are aggressive are often feared or disliked. They are not afraid to raise their voice or offend you in what they say. They often use bullying tactics to get their own way. If you are unsure how to handle this type of behaviour, ask a senior member of staff for help.

criticism: negative comments

salon scene

Sarah has been working at 'Escape' for five weeks. She really enjoys the job she is doing, especially getting to know the clients. However, one of the senior therapists is very **hostile** towards Sarah. She barks instructions at her, criticises everything she does and never praises a job well done. Yesterday, one of the clients noticed this aggressive behaviour and asked Sarah if everything was all right. Sarah is finding the senior therapist's attitude towards her very upsetting, and now that a client has noticed the problem, Sarah is starting to think that it might be best to leave the salon.

unfriendly

What do you think Sarah's next step should be?

Is leaving the best option?

How could the situation be resolved?

People, whether other staff members or clients, will react to you in the way that best fits their personality. For example, if you are aggressive, a passive person will shy away and often be offended, while an assertive person might become aggressive too. Aggressive behaviour in the salon is unprofessional.

likely to cause offence, giving a poor image of the salon

Ideally, it is good to have a mix of both passive and assertive behaviours within your personality, as this will help you to be confident and professional at work. Such a personality will also make you popular with other staff and the clients!

Dear Nat

A client came into the salon today to complain about her fake tan. She said she wasn't happy with the shade and that it looked streaky. I told her it looked fine and didn't understand why she didn't like it. She just exploded and told me to get the manager immediately, saying what did I know as I wasn't even qualified! I said to her that she had no right to talk to me like that and I would definitely get my boss over to sort her out. My boss overheard us, as the client was being a bit loud. When she had spoken to the client she said I was in the wrong and made me apologise. I am gutted and don't want to go back to work next Saturday. What should I do?

From Linzi

Nat says

Your boss is right! You should have called her over straightaway and not tried to make a judgement on behalf of the salon. You were over assertive and the client, already upset about her fake tan, became aggressive. Your boss wouldn't want the client to be upset, as this is bad for business. That is why she needed to put things right, not only with the fake tan but also with the client's feelings towards the salon staff, namely you! If you are serious about your career in the salon, then be prepared to keep your comments to yourself at this stage and let senior staff handle complaints. Go back to the salon on Saturday and put what happened down to experience. You have learned a valuable lesson.

Professional attitudes and behaviour

Salon professionalism

In the salon, you must always take care with your facial expressions and body language. You are surrounded by mirrors and do not know who might be watching! You only get one chance to make a good first impression and it is important to both the salon and your career that it is a good one.

TRY IT OUT!

Opposite is a spider diagram of positive personal behaviours. For each behaviour, write down how you have shown a good example of each – it doesn't have to be in your work in the salon, just in your behaviour generally. If you can show that you are using all the positive behaviours, then well done – you are well on your way to becoming a professional!

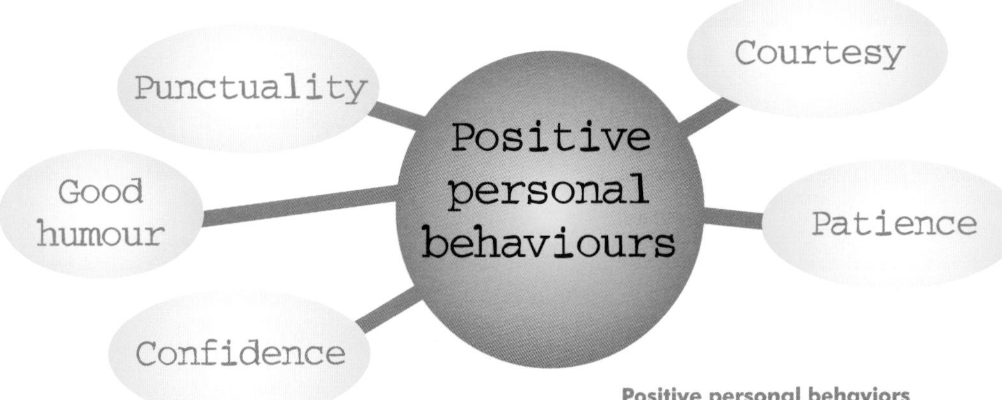

Positive personal behaviors

In the same way that positive personal behaviour will please your clients, negative behaviour will upset them and will cause problems for both you and the other salon staff. Negative publicity of any kind is never good for business. If you have created a problem by rudeness or arrogance, then this will also make you unpopular with the salon staff, as they will have to patch up the frayed relationship, forcing them to work harder on pleasing the client.

giving something a bad name

having a very high opinion of yourself

Remember that you are a valued part of the salon team. Every person in the team has a role to play in keeping clients satisfied, and your role is just as important as the manager's. By providing valuable support, such as handling payments or bookings at reception, you are one brick in the wall that builds a good strong team. Think of it like this: if you take away a brick at the bottom, what will happen to the wall?

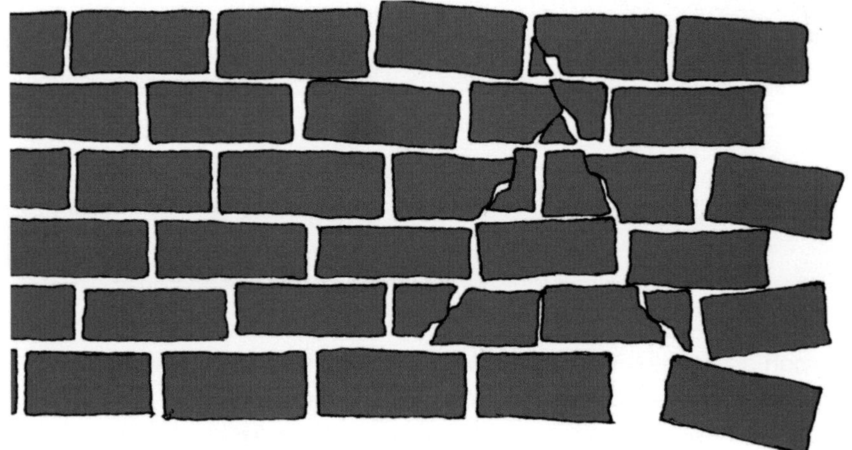

A team is like a brick wall. Take away a brick and the wall starts to crumble!

TRY IT OUT!

Has anyone ever been arrogant or bad tempered with you? Think about when you have experienced negative attitudes like these in a shop or at school. Write a short paragraph about the experience and how it made you feel. You can ask a family member or friend for their thoughts too.

salon scene

One busy Saturday, Nikita was at work in the salon and witnessed a disturbing incident. A client had come into the salon for acrylic nail extensions but had brought her 3-year-old son with her. Nikita's boss had agreed to carry out the treatment (not wanting to lose the client or the money) on the understanding that the child would play quietly. Nikita did her best to keep the child entertained, but her help was needed elsewhere in the salon. The little boy became restless and started to play with the therapist's equipment. Both his mother and the therapist told him to stop but he accidentally knocked over an open bottle of acetone and it splashed into his eye. The salon's first aider immediately rinsed the boy's eye with eye bath from the first aid kit. He was taken to hospital for further treatment.

Do you think Nikita's boss was right to allow the child to stay in the salon?

How could this situation have been avoided without both the client and the salon losing out?

How could an incident like this affect the professional reputation of the salon?

The most enjoyable part of working in a salon is doing a job you love and spending time with people you like. However, not everyone you meet will necessarily be someone you like. You will have to learn tolerance of others and how to adapt your behaviour to fit in with people of all ages, social status, ethnicity and skill levels. Look at the table of examples of good practice when dealing with different clients.

being patient

position in life

people from different cultures and/or religions

Examples of good practice when dealing with clients

Clients	Example of good practice
The elderly	Never rush them – give them time to keep up with you. Help with standing if needed. You may need to speak clearly and a little louder if their hearing is poor.
Children	Talk to them on their level and don't use confusing language. Help them when climbing onto a high chair, e.g. a styling chair.
People of different social status	You must show respect to all clients and staff whatever their status. You may find that some wealthy clients expect special treatment.
People from different ethnic groups	If you are having trouble understanding a person's accent, then ask for help from a senior member of staff. Never avoid talking to someone because it is hard to communicate with them.
People with different skill levels	You may have clients of all abilities, e.g. visually impaired or with physical disabilities. Speak to all clients politely and offer help where needed, e.g. move obstructions or read out the price list.

visually impaired: not able to see well or at all

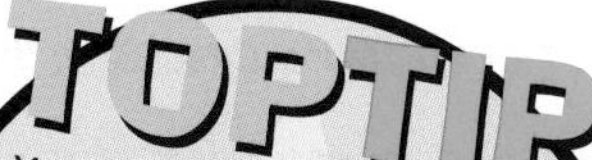

You should remain calm and in control at all times in the salon, especially when dealing with a difficult situation. Never let a client see that you are getting angry – stay professional. If you feel you cannot control your anger, then excuse yourself and find someone else to deal with the situation.

OVER TO YOU...

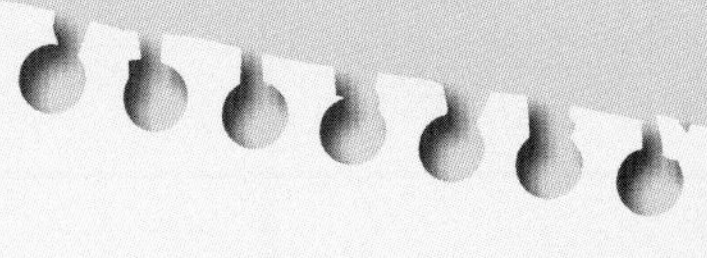

Write a short report on why people choose to go to one salon rather than another. Ask family members and friends for their reasons. Include your own experiences too.

Responding positively to constructive criticism and feedback

How can you do something right if you don't know you are doing it wrongly in the first place? Constructive criticism is when someone tells you that you are not very good at something but in a way that will help you do it better. It is never easy when someone criticises the work you do. However, this type of criticism will play an important role in your development, so you will need to be mature about it and think about how you can do a better job next time.

From time to time, you may even be asked to cast a critical eye over something yourself, and you should always give feedback that respects the person's feelings. You will be judged in the salon by both other staff and clients, and how you react to the judgements made about you is a true test of your character.

Of course, there are always people who are over critical. This type of behaviour is best ignored, or you might want to discuss it with a senior member of staff.

Dear Nat

Today, in the salon there was an argument between one of the senior stylists and her junior. One told the other that her cutting ability wasn't up to much and they had a stand-up row in the staff room but everyone could hear it on the salon floor. My boss rushed in there, told them to stop arguing and to wait until she had finished her client and was able to sort out their differences. I felt really embarrassed and didn't know where to look. I was just quiet all day after that.

From Joshua

Nat says

This type of criticism causes a negative reaction. If only the stylist had told the manager how she felt about her colleague's ability, I'm sure the manager would have suggested further training without upsetting anyone's feelings. I can understand why you were embarrassed, but you should have carried on as if nothing had happened for the rest of the day so that clients wouldn't sense an atmosphere.

The importance of confidentiality

Confidentiality is vital to maintain a positive and happy atmosphere in the salon. You need a high level of trust when dealing with sensitive information. For example, a client may not want anyone to know that she has a lip and chin wax, as facial hair on women is not socially acceptable in Britain. You have a responsibility to both the salon and clients to keep any information private, and that includes addresses and telephone numbers. There are laws about keeping information on clients confidential and you must not break them, otherwise the salon or you may be sued.

not discussing personal or sensitive information

something not liked by most people

taken to court for compensation

TRY IT OUT!

Read each of the scenarios below and on page 24 about what might happen if confidentiality is broken and answer the questions.

Scenario 1

A client asks for the telephone number of another client as she hasn't seen her for a while. You give it to her because you remember seeing them chatting in the salon in the past. A few days later, the client whose number you gave out storms angrily into the salon demanding an apology and compensation for distress. The other client has begun to make abusive phone calls to her about an issue with a family member. She informs your boss that he will be facing legal action for giving out her telephone number.

money

Do you think the client has a right to be angry? Has confidentiality been broken?

Scenario 2

While chatting to a friend you let it slip that a client, whom you both know, is pregnant but hasn't told her parents yet. You make her promise to keep the secret, but unfortunately she tells her mum who knows the client's parents. This causes a lot of trouble for the salon when the parents find out and your boss sacks you.

Do you think you have a right to discuss other people's personal lives? Have you been treated unfairly?

Scenario 3

On the bus home from the salon you are discussing with a friend an anti-cellulite treatment that a regular client has. You are both laughing about the client's 'lumpy legs'. You are unaware that the client's friend is behind you on the bus. She informs the client about your behaviour, who reports it to the salon saying that she will never return. Your boss gives you a written disciplinary warning as a result of the incident.

Do you think you have been fairly treated? In what way have you broken confidentiality?

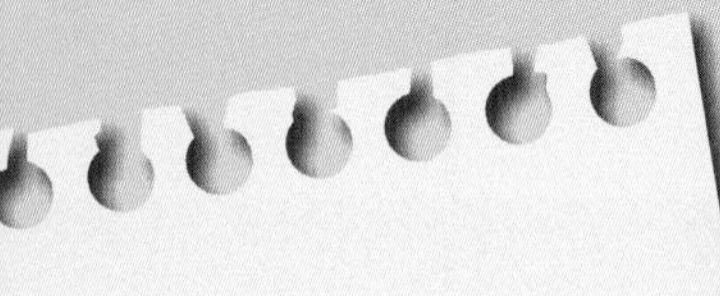

OVER TO YOU...

Now that you've looked at all aspects of customer service, ask family members or friends about their experiences of salons. When they had a good experience, what did they particularly like about the salon that made them want to return? If their experience was bad, what annoyed them and perhaps made them decide to take their business elsewhere? Think about your own experiences. Write a short report on customer service using your own experiences and the information you have gathered.

Check what you know...

Watch out! Some questions have more than one correct answer.

1. In the salon you should always speak:
   - [ ] clearly and politely
   - [ ] loudly
   - [ ] very quietly so as not to disturb people working

2. What might happen if you don't listen carefully to a client's requests?
   - [ ] they might think you understand when you don't
   - [ ] they might complain to the salon staff about you
   - [ ] they might not give you a tip

3. As a client enters the salon, what should your reaction be?
   - [ ] ignore him, after all you are busy
   - [ ] shout over that you will be there in a minute
   - [ ] greet him in a polite and friendly way and ask if you can help

4. A client becomes angry in the salon. Do you?
   - [ ] ask her to leave as she is being rude
   - [ ] stay calm and call over a senior member of staff
   - [ ] run into the staff room laughing loudly

5. You are really upset as you have had a row with your boyfriend on the way to the salon. Should you?
   - [ ] tell your boss and explain why you are upset
   - [ ] burst into tears as soon as you walk through the salon door
   - [ ] be angry with everyone all day, refusing to smile

6. You are experiencing a quiet period in the salon. What should you do?
   - [ ] sit at reception, read a magazine and have a cup of tea
   - [ ] sneak off to the staff room to pretend you are busy
   - [ ] ask other members of staff if there is anything you can do

7. You notice an elderly client struggling to open the door to come into the salon. What should you do?
   - [ ] immediately offer assistance
   - [ ] laugh
   - [ ] tell someone else as you are busy

8. The salon manager tells you that the way you dress in the salon is not appropriate. How should you react?
   - [ ] tell him that you don't like the way he dresses either
   - [ ] ask how he thinks you should dress appropriately
   - [ ] run off crying as you are trying your best

9. You overhear a private conversation in the salon about someone you know. Should you:
   - [ ] text your friend immediately that you have some great gossip for her
   - [ ] put it out of your mind, it is nothing to do with you
   - [ ] join in the conversation straight away as you know who they are talking about

10. You find a £20 note on the floor at reception. What should you do with it?
    - [ ] keep it, because you found it first
    - [ ] tell your boss straight away
    - [ ] put it in the staff tip box

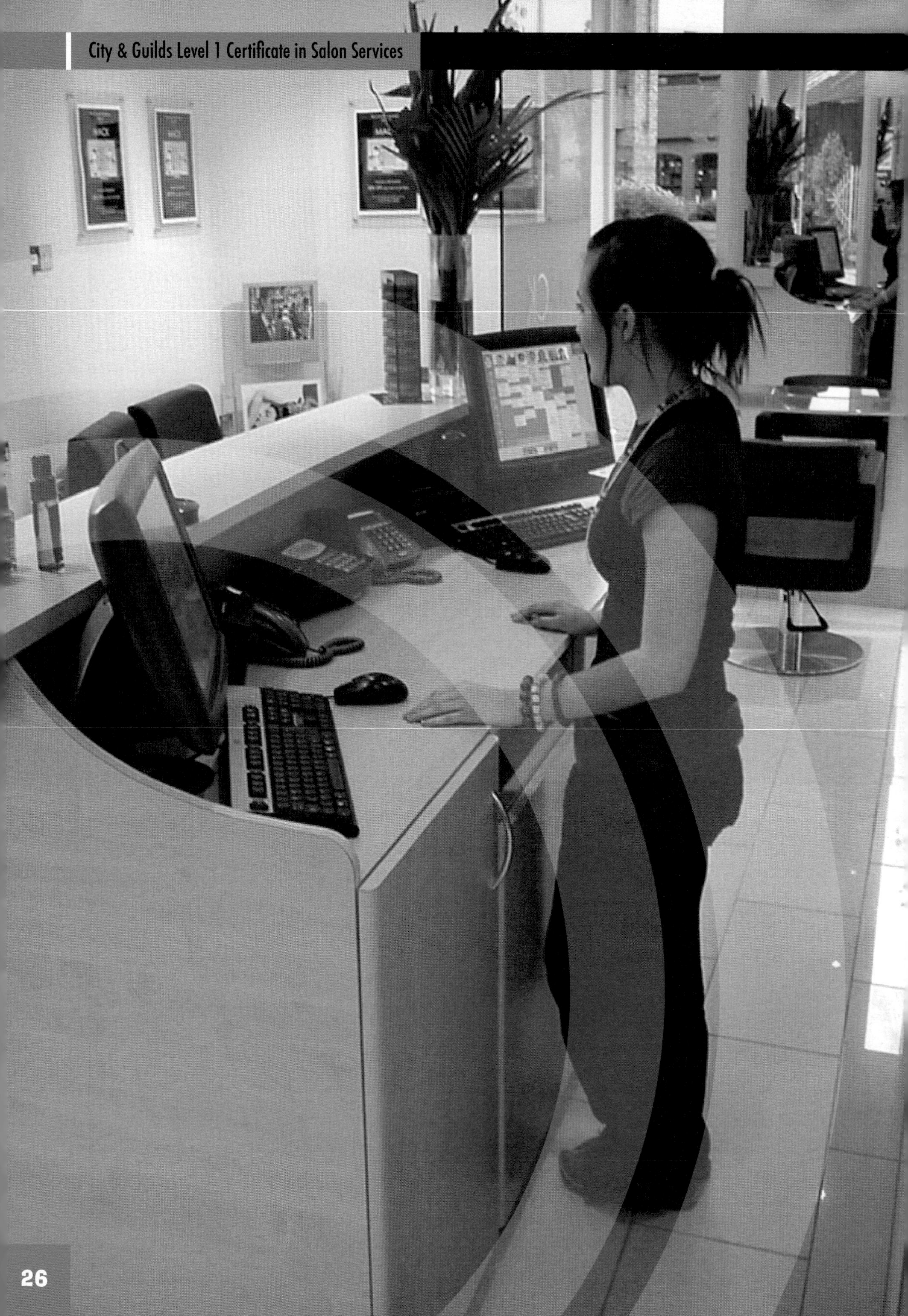

Unit 2

Salon reception

The reception area is usually the first place that clients will see when they enter the salon. As it will be their first impression of the salon, a welcoming, tidy and professional looking reception is essential. When you deal with clients at reception, you too will need to present a professional image. Remember to be friendly and welcoming and look professional at all times.

This unit links closely with Unit 1 Customer service as that is exactly what you are giving as a receptionist.

In this unit you will learn about:

- Presenting a positive personal image.
- Basic salon reception duties.
- Making appointments for salon services.
- Dealing with payments at reception.

There is no observation of your performance for this unit.

Presenting a positive personal image

The reception area and your presence in it should present a clear message to all clients:

- It must be **welcoming** – pleasing to the eye.
- It must be **tidy** – kept free from clutter at all times.
- It must look **inviting** – products and information need to be displayed professionally.
- You should look **professional** – make sure you have all the right equipment to hand such as the appointment book, telephone, pens, and so on.

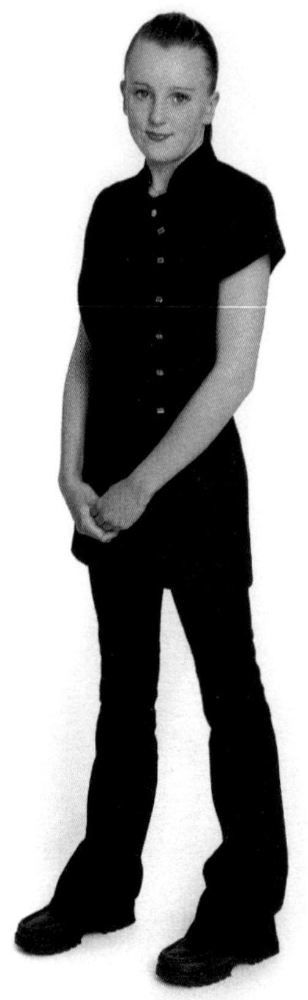

Personal presentation is very important

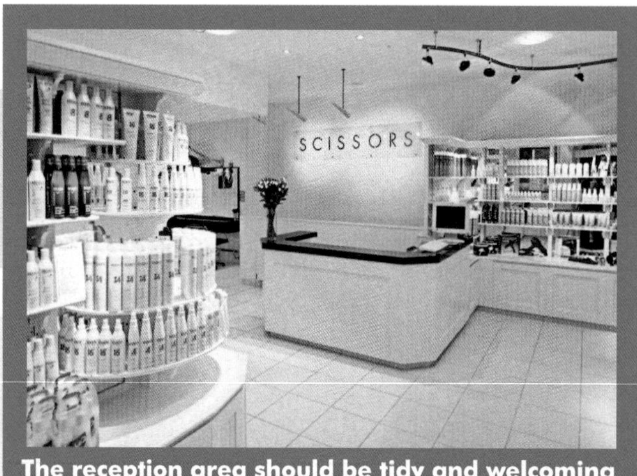

The reception area should be tidy and welcoming

items for sale

OVER TO YOU...

Think about the products that are displayed and sold at the reception area in the salon where you work. Do you think the salon provides a good retail selection?

Find out what other local salons provide. You could visit them and ask for a price list of the retail products, or ask someone you work with to take you to the wholesalers to look at the different product displays there. Remember to pick up any information you find as you go along.

Write a short report on the range of products available in the reception area of a variety of salons. Describe the ways the products are displayed. Does the type of products a salon sells have anything to do with its image? If you wish, you can include sketches, pictures from magazines, photographs or any other information you have gathered.

Personal appearance and behaviour

The way the reception area looks is only a part of what impresses clients. How you present yourself is also very important. You must be dressed smartly and professionally in the correct uniform, with your hair and make-up done to complement the look. Initially, you may need advice on how to dress and do your hair and make-up in the way that the salon prefers. Don't take this as criticism of your own style – it's about presenting the image of the salon which might involve all staff being styled in the same way.

fits in with, looks good together

However, some salons are flexible in the way the staff dress and look and may encourage individualism. This type of salon policy might influence where you would prefer to work. If you want to keep your own identity, then a salon with a strict dress code won't be for you!

looking different from everyone else

Look at the personal appearance checklist below. Each time you work in the salon, especially if you are working on reception, use the checklist to see if you are fully prepared and well presented.

Personal appearance checklist

Personal presentation	Tick ✔ if you are ready
Are you freshly bathed or showered and wearing deodorant?	
Are your teeth brushed and your breath fresh?	
Are you wearing the correct uniform?	
Is your uniform/clothing clean and ironed?	
Are you wearing appropriate make-up?	
Are you wearing the appropriate amount of jewellery?	
Is your hair well styled and tied up if necessary?	
Is your footwear appropriate and clean?	
Are your hands and nails clean and well manicured?	

You will need to work hard to provide a high level of customer service whenever you are in reception and your behaviour should be professional at all times. You should attend to clients entering the salon as soon as possible and always with a friendly greeting and a smile on your face. This can be difficult when you have had a busy day and may be feeling tired or irritable. However, this is where your level of professionalism will be tested and you must put on a happy, smiling face!

There are two golden rules to providing a professional service at reception:

- Remain calm and pleasant at all times.
- If there is something you cannot handle, ask a senior member of staff.

You will be expected to deal with a wide range of enquiries and a variety of situations. As long as you communicate in a clear and pleasant manner and stick to the two golden rules, you will find that with experience you will become more confident and professional in your approach. The spider diagram below shows the positive communication skills that you will need to have.

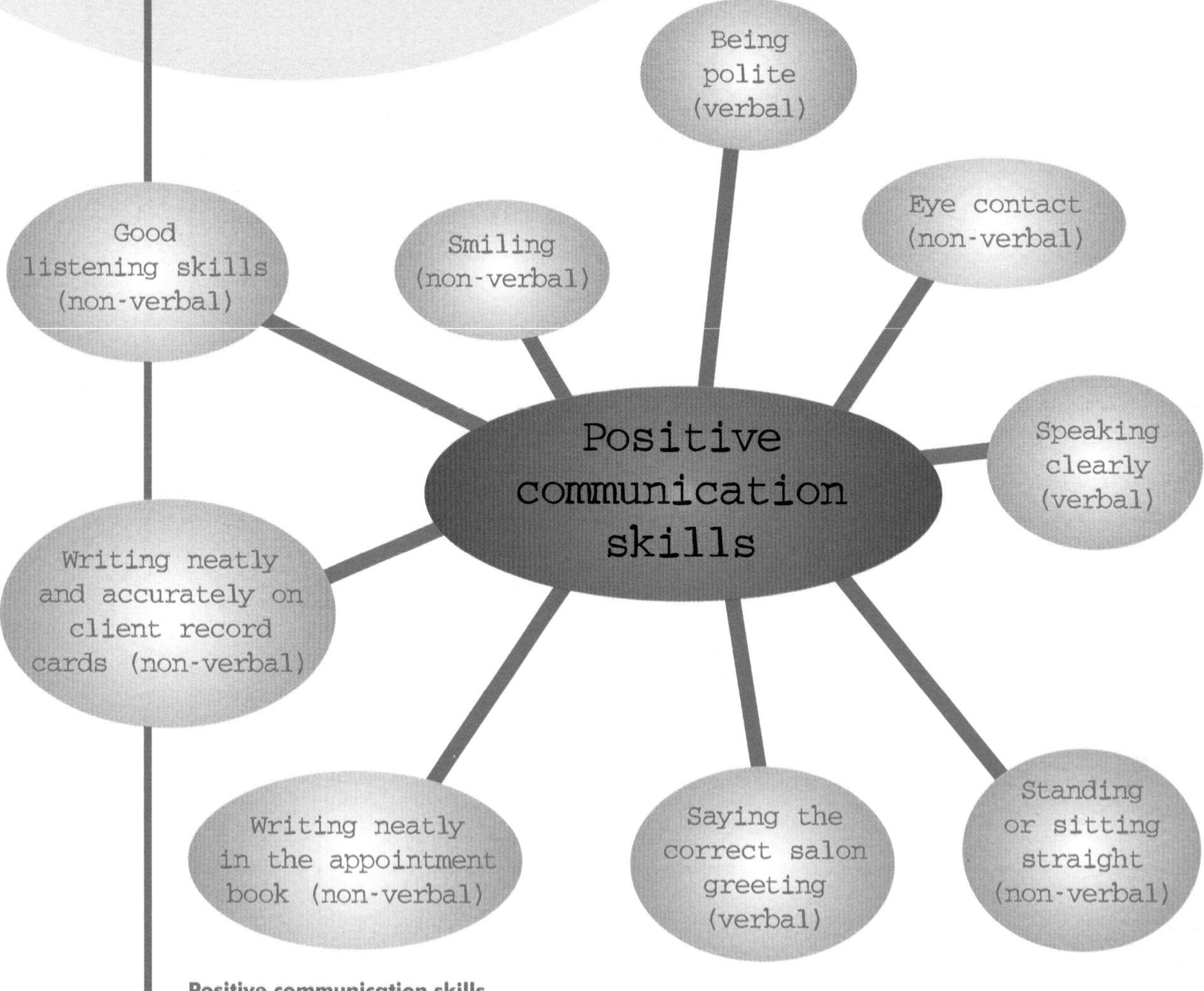

Positive communication skills

TRY IT OUT!

Look at the spider diagram of positive communication skills on page 30. Are there any others that would help you to be professional in the reception area? If so, list them. You could discuss them with other staff in the salon or your tutor.

Write down a suitable and professional greeting that could be used when dealing with a client on the telephone. (Look at the suggestion in Unit 1 Customer service on page 11 as a reminder.)

salon scene

The salon receptionist, Ayesha, had been at a party last night and arrived at work feeling a little under the weather after a late night. She looked pale and washed out and the little amount of make-up she had applied wasn't covering up the dark circles under her eyes. Her uniform was stained and creased, her hair was untidy and her breath smelled stale. All the staff were giggling about how she looked and asking her about her night out, but Ayesha's manager didn't look too pleased. She took Ayesha into the staff room and told her either to smarten herself up or go home and lose a day's pay as she felt she did not look professional enough to represent the salon at reception.

Are you surprised at the manager's reaction?

Do you think Ayesha is right to go out and have fun, knowing she has to be presentable for work the next day?

Should she have phoned in sick?

Would you have done what Ayesha did?

Basic salon reception duties

Now let's look at the basic salon reception duties you will be expected to carry out as part of your role while working on reception. These will involve:

- Receiving clients at reception.
- Offering services at reception.
- Promoting the sale of products, services and treatments.

Receiving clients at reception

When receiving clients at reception you will be expected to:

Receiving clients at reception

- Take the client's coat and offer a gown if appropriate
- Use the correct, professional salon greeting
- Check the client's appointment in the appointment book
- Take care of the client's belongings
- Seat the client comfortably in reception

How to receive clients at reception

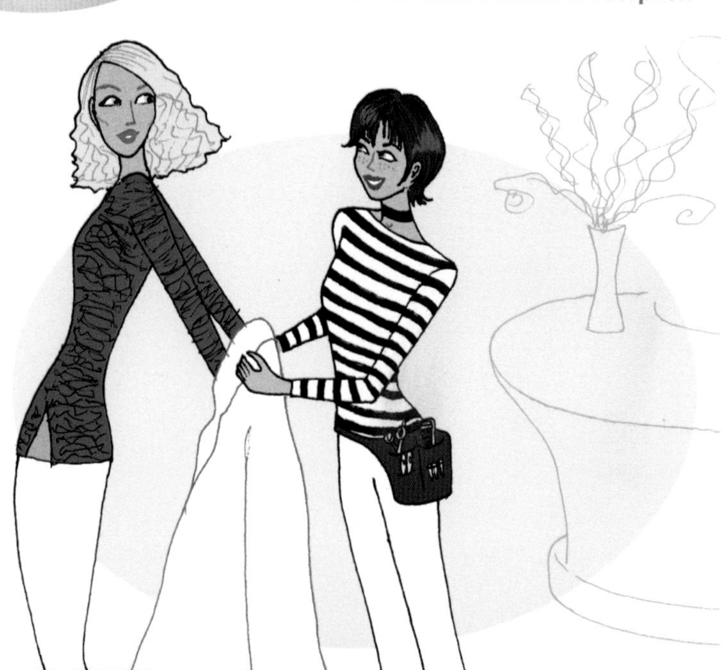

Welcome clients in a friendly and efficient way

TRY IT OUT!

Consider all the tasks in the spider diagram on page 32. Now put them in the order in which you think they should be completed. Check your order with the list below.

Your list should have looked like this:

1 Greet the client using the salon's correct professional response. You should, by now, be familiar with the importance of using the correct professional greeting.

2 Ask the client about his or her appointment and check it off in the appointment book – inform staff of the client's arrival after he or she is seated in reception.

3 Take the client's coat, hang it up and offer a gown, if appropriate.

4 Ask the client to take a seat in the reception area – consider the client's needs, e.g. is the client a wheelchair user?

5 Take care of the client's belongings – this may involve storing them at reception or in a suitable area.

Offering services at reception

Now you have received the client in a professional manner, you can begin to think about the services that you offer at reception, for example offering the client refreshment.

It is polite to ask a client if he or she would like a drink or a magazine while waiting. Even if the client is taken through into the salon immediately, you may still offer a magazine or a drink, depending on the service. For example, it would not be practical to do this if the treatment required the client to lie on a couch.

practical: suitable or sensible

Offering hot and cold drinks to clients is common practice in a salon environment. Usually the client is not charged for this as it is seen as part of the service.

You should take care with hot drinks, not only when handling them yourself but also where you place them. Make sure you put them down on a stable and safe surface where there is no risk of the drink being knocked over or spilt. Any spillages should be wiped up immediately to prevent accidents.

Next time you are in the salon's reception area, look at the range of magazines and newspapers available. They should be current – old or tatty looking magazines should be regularly removed. The type of magazines will depend on the salon's clientele. If the salon has a mix of male and female, teenage and elderly clients, for example, then there should be a suitable range of magazines and newspapers to interest everyone.

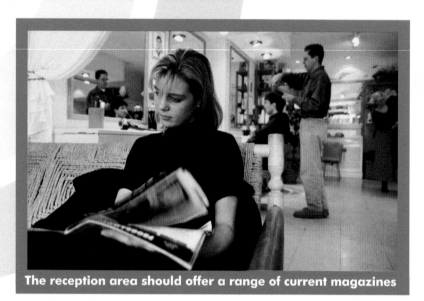

The reception area should offer a range of current magazines

Some salons go out of their way to provide a comfortable waiting area with music, a television and even a games console. Others do not consider this important and may not offer anything other than a seat.

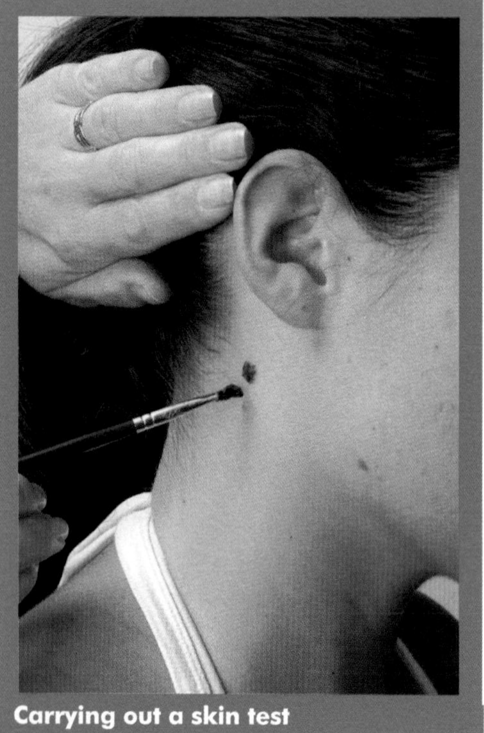

Carrying out a skin test

One other important service that may be carried out at reception is skin testing. A skin test is carried out in advance of a service that uses chemicals, such as a perm, to check whether the client is allergic to the chemicals. (If the client is allergic, then the treatment cannot take place.) The test involves mixing a little of the product to be used and dabbing it onto a small area behind the client's ear. It is a quick and easy process, but you will need training on how to do a skin test before working alone on reception.

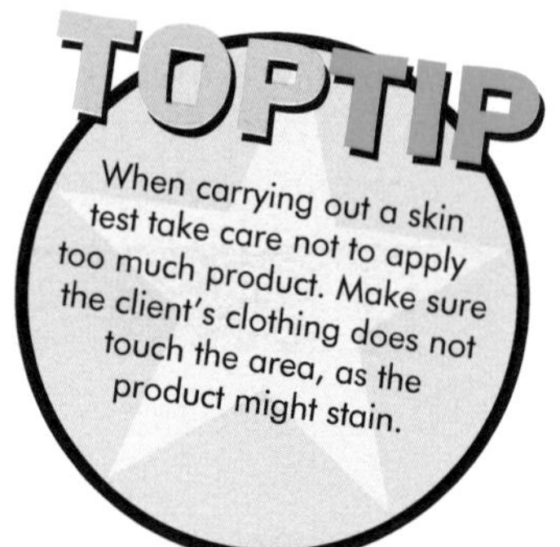

TOPTIP
When carrying out a skin test take care not to apply too much product. Make sure the client's clothing does not touch the area, as the product might stain.

OVER TO YOU...

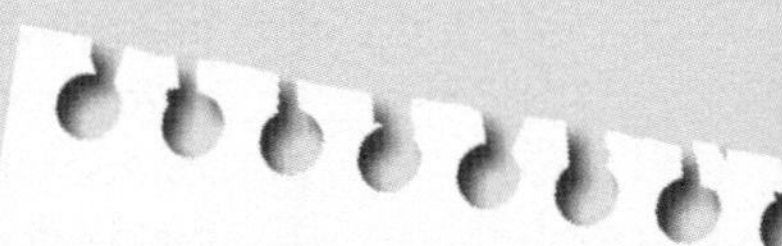

Investigate the services provided at reception in a range of salons in your area. Include a salon within a gym and a barber's as part of your research. Note the different services offered, then discuss them with friends and family. Find out their experiences of salon reception facilities and what they would like to have available whilst they wait for services or treatments. Write a short report on the services provided by salons for customers waiting in reception.

Promoting the sale of products, services and treatments

As part of your duties at reception, you may be expected to promote the products, services and treatments of the salon. You will need to be familiar with what your salon offers – if you have already completed the 'Try it out' activity on page 15, then you will have done this research. If not, do it now to help you brush up on your knowledge of the products and services of the salon.

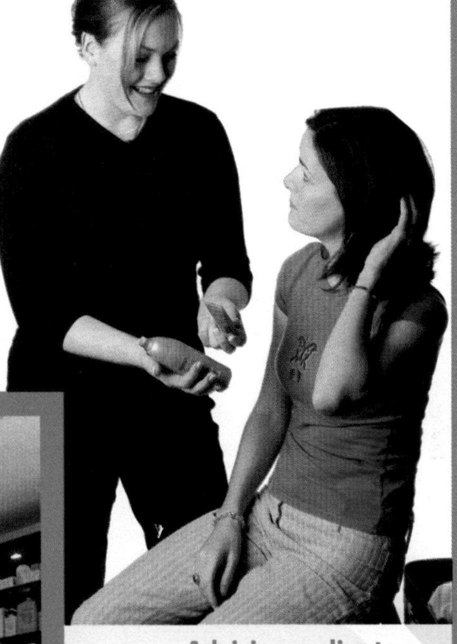

Advising a client on a suitable product

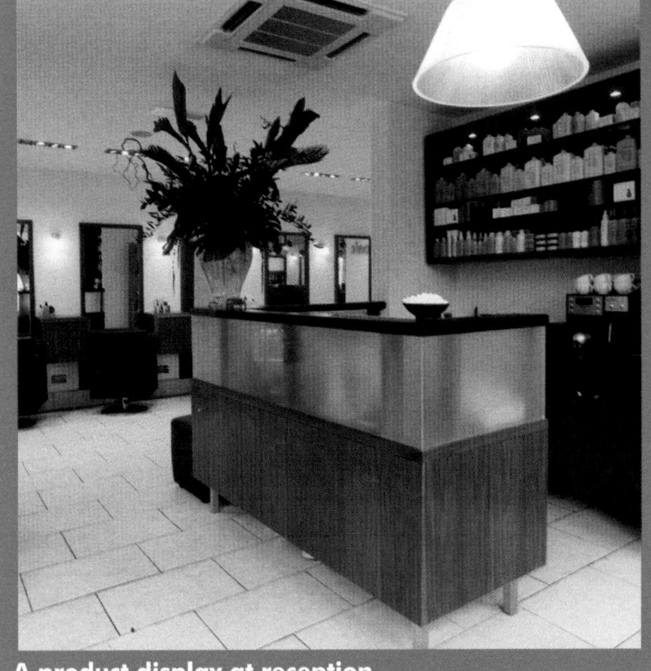

A product display at reception

Remember, when offering clients advice on products or services you are not allowed by law to mislead them in any way. To ensure the information you give is correct, always read the product label. If in doubt, ask a senior member of staff. If you are able to promote the products and services of the salon effectively, then this will show both the client and your employer that you are professional in your approach.

effectively: well and successfully

The key to confidence in promoting products, services and treatments is to understand their features and benefits – what they have to offer to a client. For example, a semi-permanent colour will add shine or tone to the hair, and this is a good selling point. Below is a table of features and benefits of some of the treatments and services that your salon may provide.

Features and benefits of various treatments and services

Treatment/service	Features and benefits
Cutting	Removes split or dead ends; offers a new style/ reshape to hair
Perming	Permanently adds wave or curl to hair
Colouring	Adds shine or tone to hair, covers grey hair, highlights hair colour; can be permanent or non-permanent
Waxing	Removes unwanted hair (must be longer than 2 mm in length); can take up to five weeks to grow back
Manicure	Shapes nails and improves condition of hands and nails
Facial	Exfoliates the skin, adds moisture and gives the skin a fresh appearance

Exfoliates: removes dead skin cells

TRY IT OUT!

Look at the above table of features and benefits of various services and treatments. Now, try writing a table of features and benefits for the products offered by the salon where you work.

Dear Nat

Last week, a company rep came into the salon to give us all some training on a new product range we have just launched. Then today, I advised a client about the benefits of the product range on her skin and she bought both a cleanser and moisturiser. I felt really good about the way I handled the sale and although I was nervous, I felt confident when talking to the client about the products we sell. I remembered what the rep said and tried to use her words when explaining the benefits. It really worked! My boss was pleased with me and praised me to all the other staff. I can't wait to use these selling skills again and won't feel as nervous next time.

From Jay

Nat says

Well done! You have taken on board everything you learned from the technical rep and used it to good effect. If you have a good product knowledge, then there is no need to lack confidence in promoting the products of your salon and I'm sure you have set a good example for all the staff at the salon.

OVER TO YOU...

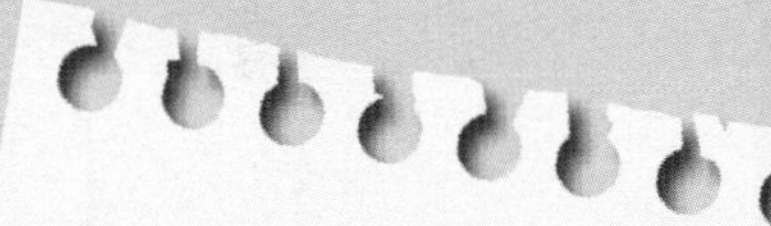

In what ways do salons provide information about their services and treatments? Collect brochures, business cards, flyers and so on, from a range of salons. You could also ask family members and friends how they decide what services to have. Write a short report on what you have found out.

Making appointments for salon services

You will be given training before you are expected to deal with the salon's appointment system – it is important that you feel confident and understand how it works. Take time to work alongside the salon staff while they are running the reception area to allow you to learn how to make appointments correctly. There are three things to consider when making appointments for clients:

- What information do you require from the client?
- What type of appointment recording system does the salon use?
- What is the duration and cost of services and treatments?

time/length

Information required from the client

Each time you make an appointment for a client, you will need to find out exactly what service or treatment he or she requires. Follow the five-step process below to help you get the right information.

TOP TIP

Don't forget to smile when taking an appointment over the telephone, as the caller will hear this in the tone of your voice and it will present a friendly image.

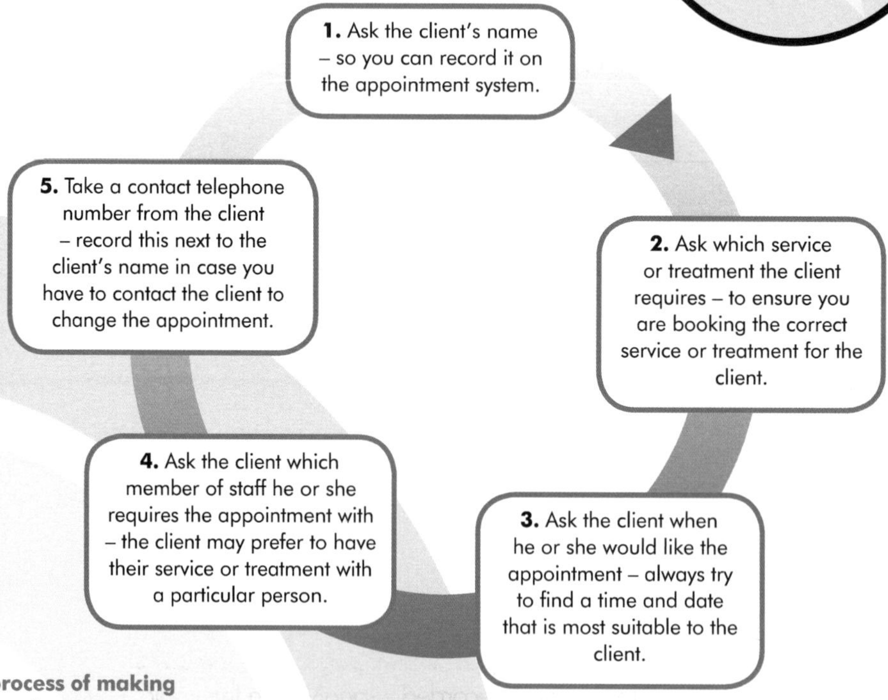

1. Ask the client's name – so you can record it on the appointment system.

2. Ask which service or treatment the client requires – to ensure you are booking the correct service or treatment for the client.

3. Ask the client when he or she would like the appointment – always try to find a time and date that is most suitable to the client.

4. Ask the client which member of staff he or she requires the appointment with – the client may prefer to have their service or treatment with a particular person.

5. Take a contact telephone number from the client – record this next to the client's name in case you have to contact the client to change the appointment.

The process of making an appointment

Appointment recording systems

There are two methods of recording information for appointments:

- A written system.
- An electronic system.

Written system

A written recording system consists of an appointment book which is set out in columns. Each member of staff has their own column and every column is divided into appropriately spaced timings, usually 15 minutes. Look at the examples of pages from a beauty appointment book and a hairdressing appointment book.

DATE 18th June – Monday
STYLISTS 1 2 3 4 5 6
8 9 10 11 12 1 2 3 4 5 6 7 8
00 15 30 45
Leah
Mrs Taylor
01211 400100
P/W
Nent
C/B/D
P/W
Mrs Rahim
W/CUT
LUNCH
Mrs Westerby
01233 497777
Hi-lights (top)
Mr Westerby
01422 620997
D/TR
Rinse
C/B/D
Hi-lights
Mrs Champion
07908 317194
Re-growth colour
Mrs Pattell
07960 062154
C/B/D
Andrew
Mrs Dodds
01233 201958
S/S
Mrs Potts
01422 150993
Semi-Colour
C/O S/S
Rinse
C/B/D
colour
LUNCH
Mrs Moorman
01211 955643
full head
foils x 2 colours
Rinse
Restyle
colour
Rinse
C/B/D
colour
Mrs Palmer
cancellation required
with Nicola after
3pm for wet cut
Shelly
Mr Davies
01211 4522111
TR
Mrs Singh
01211 412121
Mr Rees
01211 514512
flat top
Danni
Graham
x 2 TRIMS
Mr O'Hara
C/B/D
LUNCH
Tedore
long hair
S/S
C/B/D +
hair up
Mrs Adam
01211 290094
B/dry

Page from a hairdressing appointment book

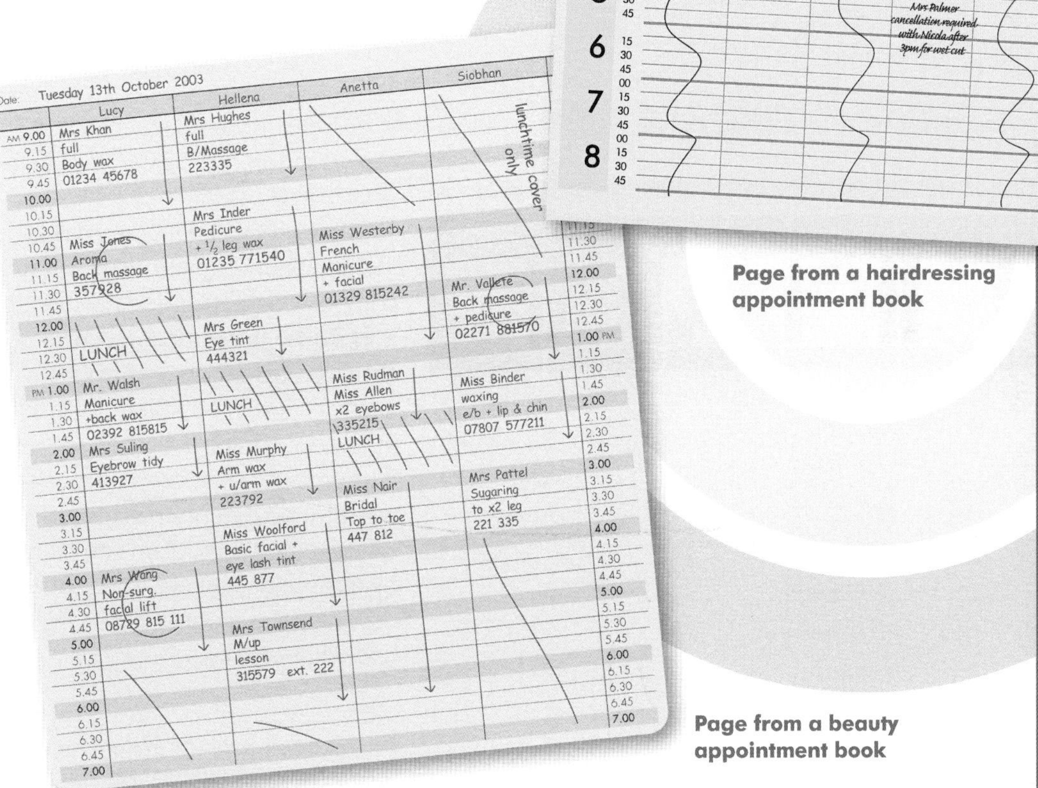

Page from a beauty appointment book

There is a lot of information recorded on an appointment page so it must be accurate, up to date and legible. The appointment page plans the day's work for the staff and if the information is recorded wrongly, then this could throw the whole salon day into chaos.

legible: clear and easy to read

Always check with a senior member of staff before entering information into the appointment system, as this will ensure that you are not responsible for mistakes that are made.

Appointment time is incorrect
- You may have to cancel the appointment and so lose money!
- The client may be kept waiting

Client has been entered for the wrong service
- Presents an unprofessional image which could damage the salon's reputation
- The client will be disappointed if they cannot have the service they want

Client's appointment is not recorded on the appointment system
- The client will be disappointed if you cannot carry out the service
- Presents an unprofessional image which could damage the salon's reputation

What could happen if the appointment page contains errors

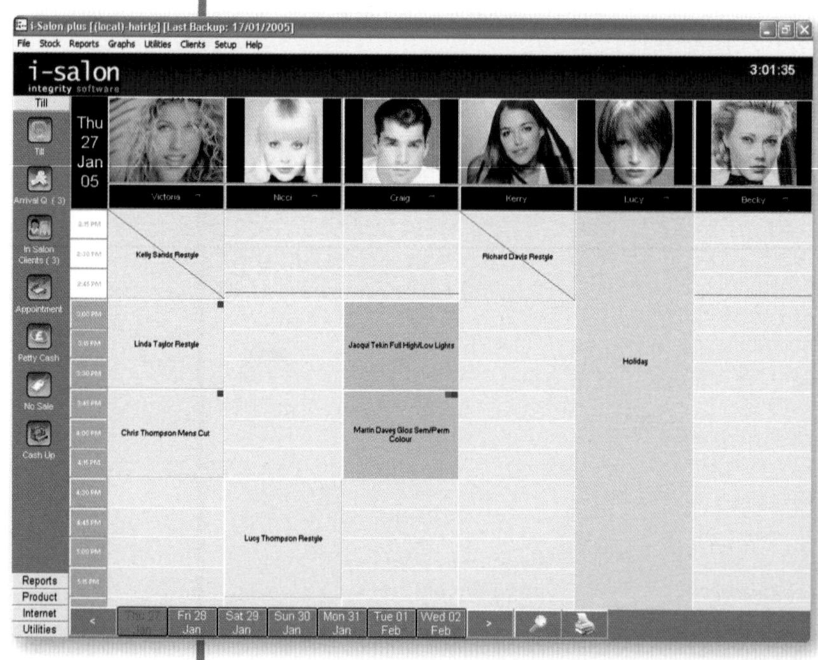

An electronic booking system (source: i-salon computer system from Integrity Software)

Electronic system

An electronic system records all the appointment information on a computer database. The advantage is that extra information, such as client contact details or previous treatments, can be stored alongside the booking information. However, if the computer goes down, the salon will have no access to its appointment system until the problem can be fixed by a support engineer. This is one advantage of a paper-based (written) booking system.

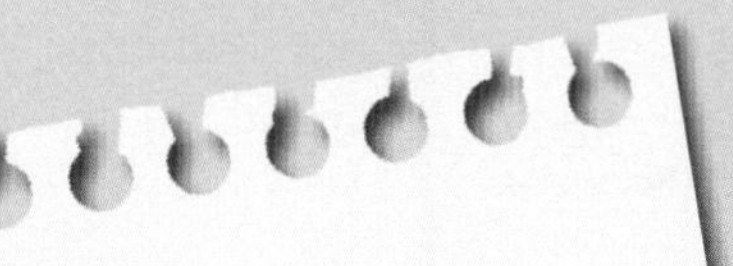

OVER TO YOU...

Visit a range of salons in your area to find out what system they use to record appointments. Ask them why they chose that particular method. Write a short report on what you have found out.

Duration and cost of services and treatments

When you are agreeing appointment times with the client, you will need to know the range of services and treatments your salon offers and the duration and cost of each. (Look back at the 'Try it out' activity you completed on page 15 which lists this information. Remember to keep your list up to date!)

Most salons have similar duration times for services and treatments, but they may differ slightly. The table (right) gives a general guide to a few of these, but you will need to find out exactly what the duration times and costs are for the salon where you work. Once you have agreed an appointment time and date with the client, double check that they know how long the appointment will take to complete. This will prevent any misunderstanding which could result in a dissatisfied client.

Duration of popular services/treatments

Service/treatment	Duration
Cut and blow dry	1 hour
Perm	2–3 hours
Re-growth colour	2 hours
Facial	1 hour
Pedicure	45 minutes
Electrolysis	15 minutes

When booking appointments, you need to understand correct appointment spacing. For example, a 15-minute slot will use one row on the appointment page, a 30-minute slot will use two rows and a 45-minute slot will use three rows. Look back at the examples of appointment pages to help you understand (page 39).

There will also be opportunities for staff to complete other services or treatments when waiting for development of colours or perms. For example, you may book a client in for a colour treatment. The consultation and application for this should take about 30 minutes, but if the colour will take 45 minutes to develop, then another service can be carried out. This is effective use of the stylist's time and is common practice in most salons, as it allows the stylist to complete more clients in a day and so bring more money into the salon. You will need to be shown how your salon's system works so that you don't over book a stylist or therapist with clients!

Taking messages

While working on reception you will be expected to take messages and pass them onto the right person. There will always be a good reason why the staff member required cannot deal with the enquiry themselves, for example they may be with a client or out on a lunch break. If you cannot pass the message on straight away, you should make a written record of the message, completing a message slip like the one shown.

MESSAGE

FOR *Deepak*

FROM *Mrs Alessi*

TEL. NO. *0208 321 145*

TELEPHONED ☑ PLEASE RING ☑

CALLED TO SEE YOU ☐ WILL CALL AGAIN ☐

WANTS TO SEE YOU ☐ URGENT ☐

MESSAGE: *Needs to speak to you asap – you can call her on the tel. no. above up to 5.30pm*

DATE: *10.05.06* TIME: *9.03am*

RECEIVED BY: *Amber*

Make sure you fill in all the details on a message slip

It is very important that all the information in a message is written out neatly, so the reader can clearly understand it. You should also make sure that you take all the information and don't forget to ask something that would be vital to the understanding of the message.

very important

It will be your responsibility once you have taken a message to ensure that it is passed on as soon as possible to the right person. If you are only in the salon one day per week and will not see that person, then you must pass the message onto another staff member who will.

salon scene

One busy Saturday, while working on reception, you take an important message for the salon manager, Jenny, as she is taking a day off. A client wishes to inform her that she won't be able to make an appointment for a practice wedding hair and make-up which she had booked for one evening the following week. As the appointment isn't written in the book and you are very busy dealing with another client, you forget to write down the message and pass it on.

Next week, when you arrive in work, Jenny is furious with you and wants to give you a formal warning. She went to the client's house along with the salon therapist only to find the client had already rung the salon to cancel! This had been a waste of time for both members of staff and did not present a very professional image to the client. You apologise and try to explain about how busy you were and that you completely forgot to take note of the message and pass it on. Jenny decides to give you another chance to prove yourself as you apologise immediately and appear very sorry for your mistake.

What can you do to ensure this situation will not happen again?

Do you think that because you apologised immediately this helped Jenny to calm down and give you another chance?

What could have happened if you had not shown any remorse for your mistake?

feeling regretful and guilty

Dealing with payments at reception

The type of payments handled through reception will differ depending on the salon where you work. The most common payment types are cash, cheques and credit/debit cards. However, your salon might also use cash alternatives such as vouchers and, if the salon is based within a hotel, clients' bills might be paid to account. Look at the table below which explains the different methods of payment.

Methods of payment

Method of payment	How it is used
Cash	Money is the most common form of payment dealt with at reception. Checking for forgeries is very important especially with larger bank notes (£20 and £50).
Cheque	This should be accompanied by a valid cheque guarantee card (which can also be used as a debit card). When paid into the bank the amount will transfer to the salon's account. Both the cheque and the guarantee card should be checked for any mistakes, e.g. has the cheque been filled out correctly and signed by the client or has the card expired?
Debit card	This is used to transfer money electronically from a person's bank account to the salon's account. A debit card may also be used as a cheque guarantee card. If the chip and pin method is not being used, then the signature on the back of the card must be checked against the client's signature to ensure that they match.
Credit card	Not all salons (especially small or medium-sized businesses) offer credit card payment as the salon will have to set up an account with the credit card company. When the card is used the credit card company agrees to make payment to the salon for the amount charged.
Vouchers	Not all salons offer gift vouchers, but they are a good alternative to offer to clients who wish to purchase a gift. They can vary in amount from £1, £5, £10 or more and can usually be used to pay for anything that the salon provides including products.
To account	If your salon is based in a hotel, then clients might charge the service, treatment or product to their hotel account. This means that whatever they spend with you in the salon is put onto their final hotel bill. This is then paid as one payment when they leave the hotel.

Although at this stage of your training, you will not be expected to handle payments at reception, you still need to be familiar with the different ways of accepting payment. While working on reception, it is a good idea to take note of how payments are handled.

Dear Nat

Today in the salon I was taking a credit card payment from a client when I noticed that the date on the card had expired. Everyone was busy and I really didn't know what to say to the client and would have felt embarrassed refusing the card, so I just took it anyway. I thought that if the payment didn't go through I would tell my boss that I didn't notice it. I know this was wrong, but how should I have handled it?

From Elycia

Nat says

Oh dear, you could have lost your salon a lot of money! If you didn't feel able to query the expired card with the client, then you should have called over a senior member of staff, preferably the salon owner or manager, and let them handle it. You did well to spot the error on the card in the first place, but then unfortunately you handled the situation wrongly. In future, no matter how busy the salon is, if there is a problem with payment, always ask a senior member of staff to deal with it.

Check what you know...

Watch out! Some questions have more than one correct answer.

1. Why must you always look presentable when working on reception?
- [ ] you will be the first person representing the salon that a client is likely to see
- [ ] in case you meet someone famous
- [ ] to present a professional image of the salon

2. Why must you keep the reception area clean and tidy?
- [ ] to keep you busy all day long
- [ ] so that the client finds the environment welcoming and pleasant
- [ ] to prevent you from breaking any laws

3. Why should you attend to enquiries as soon as possible at reception?
- [ ] to pass the time quicker
- [ ] so that you can take a client's money as quickly as possible
- [ ] so that the reception area doesn't look untidy

4. Why should you always communicate clearly and in a pleasant manner at reception?
- [ ] to show that the salon is a professional one with high standards
- [ ] to ensure that clients can understand you and are welcomed appropriately by you
- [ ] to present a professional image of the salon

5. Why do salons offer seating to clients who are waiting at reception?
- [ ] so that they don't become bored
- [ ] to use up empty space at the front of the salon
- [ ] to keep them as comfortable and happy as possible while they wait

6. Why is it good practice to offer clients a magazine and drink while they wait at reception?
- [ ] to keep them as comfortable and happy as possible while they wait
- [ ] in case they haven't had lunch
- [ ] to prevent them from becoming angry with you because you are running late

7. Why is it important to display retail products in an eye-catching way at reception?
- [ ] to ensure that clients notice them
- [ ] to try to sell as many retail products as possible
- [ ] because many other salons do it

8. When making an appointment at reception, what information would you request from a client?
- [ ] the client's name
- [ ] the client's date of birth
- [ ] the service required

9. Why must you write out a message accurately?
- [ ] to practise your handwriting
- [ ] to show you're good at filling in message slips
- [ ] to ensure the person can read and understand the message clearly

10. What is the most common form of payment made for services, treatments or products?
- [ ] cheque
- [ ] vouchers
- [ ] cash

Unit 3

Personal presentation

Personal presentation is very important when you are working in a salon environment. Clients will make judgements about the salon by the way you look, so you should always be dressed and presented in a way that will promote a professional image and make the clients feel they want to come into your salon.

In this unit you will learn about:

- The importance of a good personal image and presentation.
- Ways to encourage personal well-being.
- Ways to ensure a good personal appearance.

Towards the end of the course, you will be observed and assessed on:

- Your personal well-being.
- Your personal appearance.

The importance of a good personal image and presentation

Salon image

These days there are many different types of salon around. They range from the very funky and trendy salons to the more traditional salons, with all the others in between. A salon's image is usually aimed at the type of clients it is trying to attract, for example funky, trendy salons are more likely to attract younger clients than those where most of the clients are elderly.

One of the most important things to remember is that the image of any salon must be that of a clean, tidy and well-run salon. Your first impression when you go into a salon will help you to make your mind up whether you would want to be a client (or member of staff) there. If the salon appears to be clean, tidy and run efficiently you are likely to think it is nicer than somewhere that appears to be dirty or untidy!

being organised and not wasting time

When you are looking for work in a salon, you need to make sure the salons you are looking at can give you what you want and be a place where you will feel happy and comfortable working.

OVER TO YOU...

Describe the kind of salon you think you would like to work in, and give your reasons.

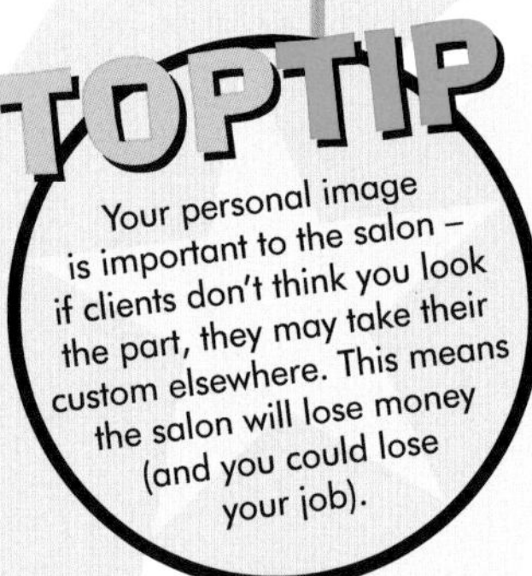

TOPTIP
Your personal image is important to the salon – if clients don't think you look the part, they may take their custom elsewhere. This means the salon will lose money (and you could lose your job).

Your personal image

First impressions are very important. People can either like or dislike you within a few minutes of your meeting because they will judge you on the way you look and the way you behave. Imagine how clients would feel if you arrived at the salon where you work looking like you had just fallen out of bed! Do you think they would want you to do their hair or beauty treatment if you looked like you could not take care of your own appearance?

The way you look matters. However good your hairdressing or beauty therapy skills may be, if you look untidy and unwashed, the image you present will give clients the wrong impression.

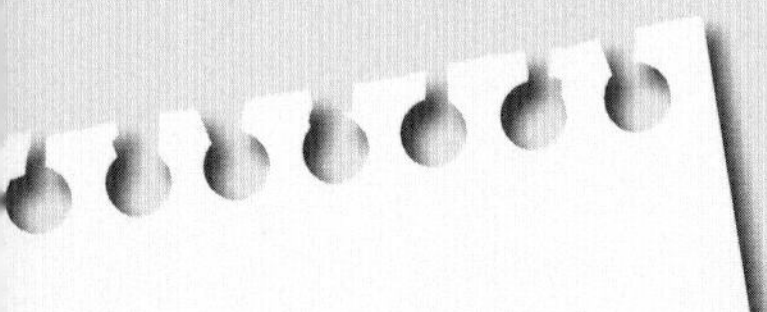

OVER TO YOU...

Collect pictures from magazines, trade catalogues, and so on, showing the different ways that staff may look when working in the salon. Include pictures of dress, uniforms, hairstyles and make-up.

Ways to encourage personal well-being

Both hairdressing and beauty therapy are demanding jobs that need lots of energy and stamina to make sure you can get through the day. It is really hard to work well when you are tired and lethargic or you are ill.

strength and staying power

have no energy

A good health routine

It is very important that you do all the things that will help you to stay fit and well, so you can do your job to the best of your ability. You need to make sure you:

- Eat a well-balanced diet.
- Have good posture when you are working.
- Take regular exercise.
- Have enough sleep.
- Take the time to relax.
- Learn how to cope with stress.

A well-balanced diet

To make sure you remain fit and healthy, you will need to eat a well-balanced diet which contains something from each of the food groups (see spider diagram).

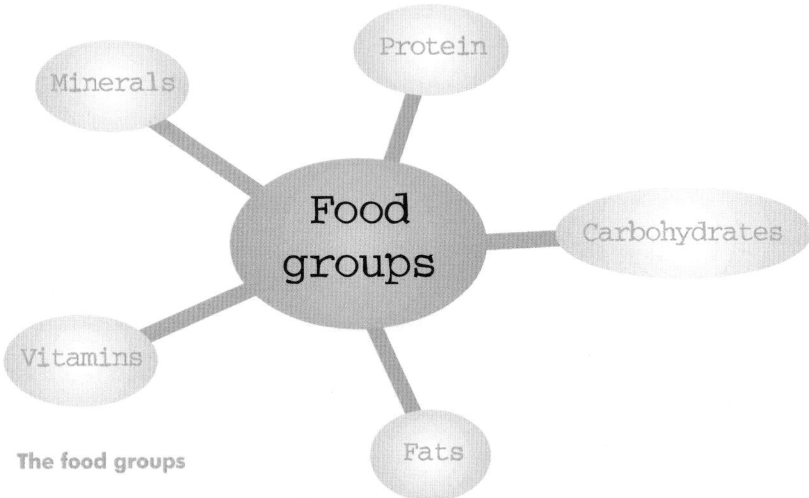

The food groups

Each of these food groups is important for different reasons. The table on page 50 looks at some of the most important components of a well-balanced diet and explains why they are important.

a part of something

Components of a well-balanced diet

Component	Where it comes from	Why it is important
Protein	Eggs, meat, fish, milk and cheese. Also in peas, beans, soya beans and nuts	It helps to build new cells in the body, e.g. hair, skin and nail cells.
Carbohydrates	Potatoes, bread and cereals. Also in sugar, jam and syrup	It provides energy.
Fats	Butter, cream, cheese, chocolate, cakes and crisps	It provides energy, but if you have too much the fat is stored in the body.
Vitamin A	Dairy products, carrots, liver and oily fish, e.g. mackerel	It keeps your eyes and skin healthy.
Vitamin B	Cereals, meat and liver	It helps the body to get energy from carbohydrates.
Vitamin C	Oranges, blackcurrants and green vegetables	It helps the body to absorb iron.
Vitamin D	Dairy food, e.g. milk, cheese, yoghurt. It is also made in the skin by the action of sunlight on the skin	It helps to build strong teeth and bones.
Calcium	Milk, cheese and other dairy products	It helps to build strong teeth and bones.
Iron	Liver, egg yolks and green vegetables	It helps to produce red blood cells.

TRY IT OUT!

Using the table above, plan a whole day's meals making sure you choose something from each food group.

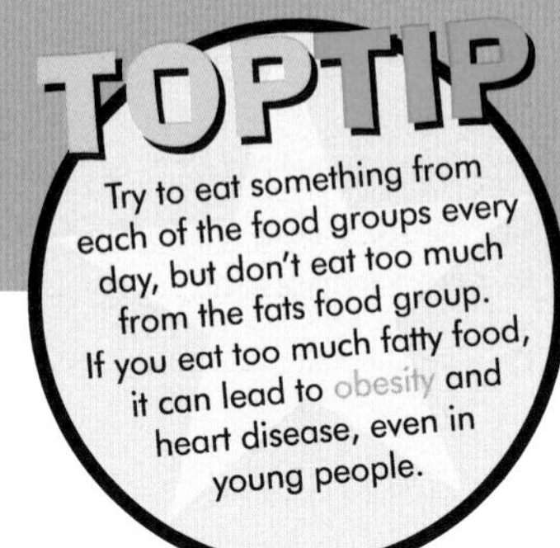

TOPTIP
Try to eat something from each of the food groups every day, but don't eat too much from the fats food group. If you eat too much fatty food, it can lead to obesity and heart disease, even in young people.

being seriously over weight

Good posture

The body you were born with has to last you a lifetime, so it is very important to look after it properly. Many hair stylists and beauty therapists suffer with back problems as a result of bad posture when working, for example stooping or leaning over the client. This is most common in taller people. In the hairdressing salon it is a good idea to use hydraulic chairs, which can be adjusted to the right height to make sure you are working comfortably.

chairs that can be moved up and down

In the beauty salon, hydraulic couches and chairs can be used, although it is better to use special beauty therapist's chairs as these have a back support, whereas a stool does not support the back. Couches and chairs should be adjusted to the right height so you can work comfortably without stooping or stretching.

As you may have to stand for long periods, you will need to make sure you are standing properly, with your weight evenly distributed.

> Keep your tools and equipment close to where you are working so you will not need to reach or stretch for things. This will prevent unnecessary stress and strain on your body and prevent injuries (like back, shoulder or neck problems).

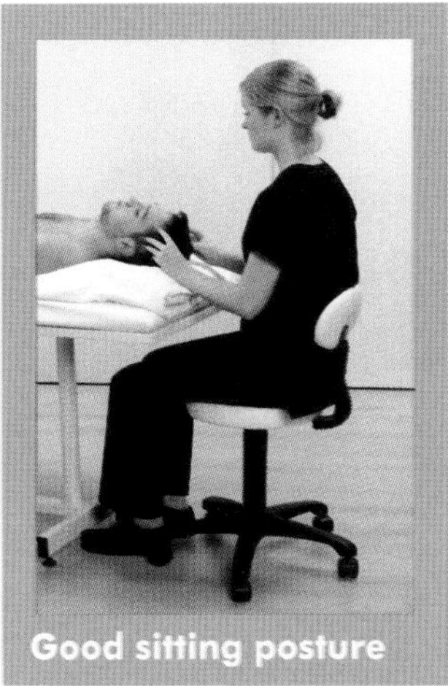
Good sitting posture

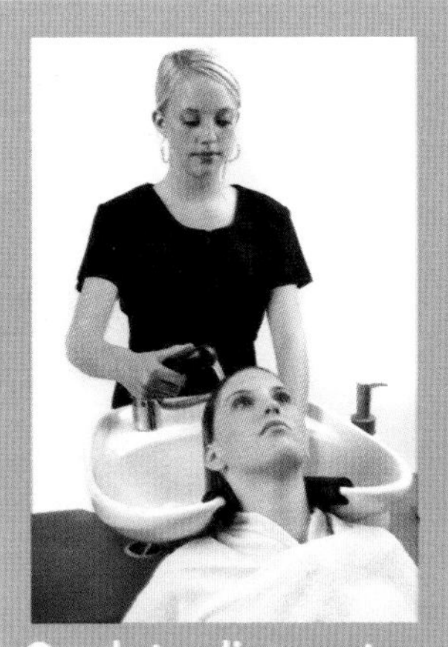
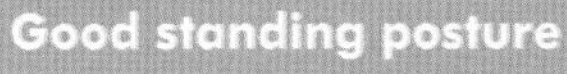
Good standing posture

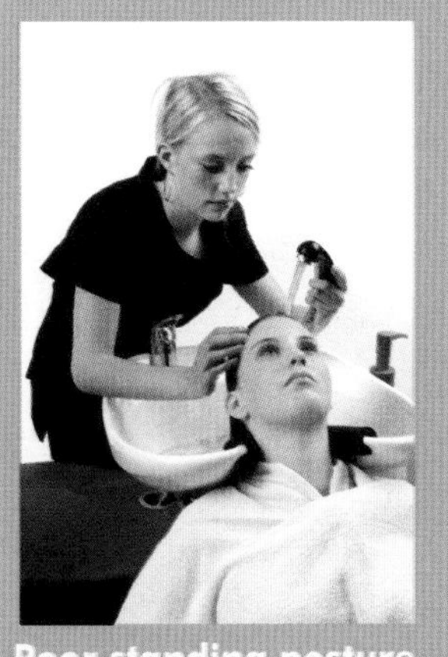
Poor standing posture

Regular exercise

You've probably heard many times how exercise is 'good for you' but did you know that it can actually help you to feel good too? If you get the right amount of exercise, it can increase your energy levels. Exercise benefits every part of the body, including the mind. It may help you sleep better, so you will feel more refreshed and awake the next day. Exercising can help you look better, too. It helps to burn calories and keeps the body looking toned.

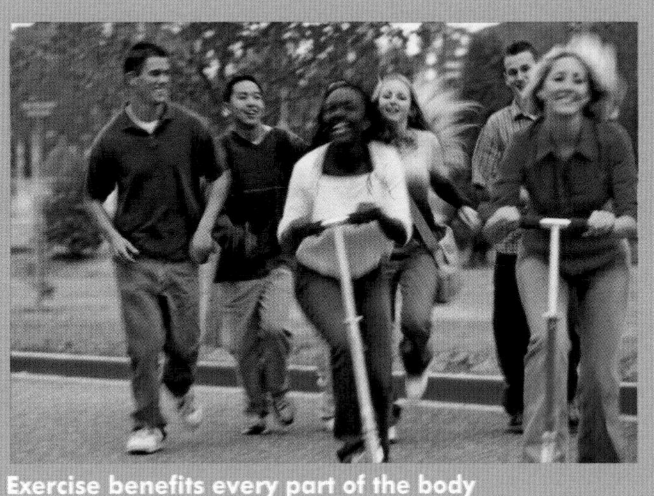
Exercise benefits every part of the body

Are you getting enough sleep?

There are no hard and fast rules about how much sleep you need – it is an individual thing. Some people need eight to ten hours' sleep per night while others need only six or seven. So how do you know how much is enough? If you have had enough sleep, you should wake up naturally and feel alert and ready to start the day. If you wake up feeling sluggish, you probably haven't had enough sleep. Sleep is important as your body repairs itself while you are asleep.

Learn to relax!

Relaxation is necessary for everyone, especially with the busy lives most people lead. You need to have time for yourself and learn to relax. You should be able to feel your muscles relax, especially the muscles in the neck and shoulders as this is where most hair stylists and beauty therapists seem to carry tension. A good way to learn to relax is by doing exercise like yoga.

muscle tightness and strain

When you feel stressed it can be difficult to deal with problems because they just seem too big. Once you have relaxed, you will find you can think things through in a clear and logical way and then work out solutions to the problems.

orderly

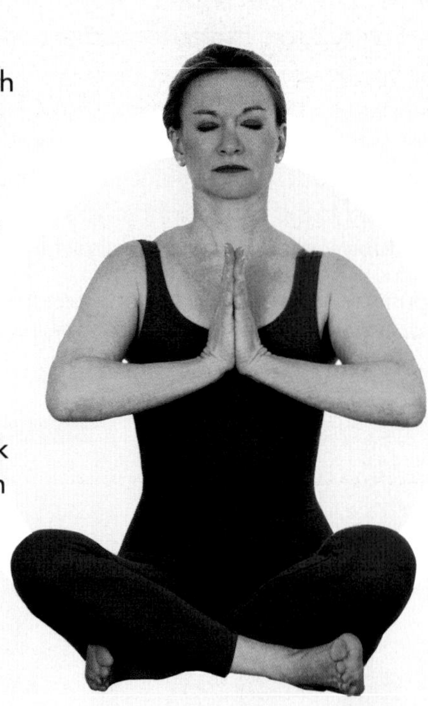

Yoga is a good way to learn to relax

Coping with stress

Most people have stress in their lives, but the important thing is knowing how to deal with stress before it gets too much for us to cope with. The first thing you must do is to decide exactly what it is in your life that is causing you to be stressed. Different things cause stress for different people. You may find you become stressed during exams, whereas someone else might be stressed at the thought of going somewhere new for the first time.

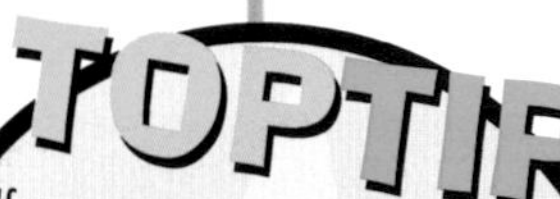

TOP TIP

If you want to try deep breathing, lie on your back with your hands on your stomach and breathe in deeply through your nose until you can't breathe in any more. Hold your breath for a few seconds and then breathe out slowly through your mouth. Try and do this for three or four breaths a few times each day.

Once you know what is causing the stress, you need to find positive ways to deal with it. Probably the easiest relaxation technique to try is deep breathing which can help to relax tense muscles and put energy to good use.

Being able to cope with stress is an important part of being a hair stylist or beauty therapist as there will be times when a stressful situation arises and you have to stay calm. These situations may include dealing with a difficult client or running late with your appointments.

salon scene

Shamecca was training to be a beauty therapist and loved working with her clients. However, every Wednesday morning her regular 10 o'clock client would usually turn up 15 minutes late for her manicure appointment. This meant that Shamecca was running behind for the rest of the morning and usually had to catch up the time during her lunch break, which meant she didn't have one.

Shamecca would wake up every Wednesday morning and start to feel stressed. She knew that all her clients that came in after 10 am would be moaning because she kept them waiting every week. Sometimes they didn't say anything, but she could tell by the way they looked at her that they weren't happy. To make matters worse, she would be starving when she finished work because she hadn't eaten. Shamecca was finding it harder and harder each week to be nice to the clients because she knew she was going to have an awful day.

What could Shamecca do to stop this stressful situation from happening every week?

OVER TO YOU...

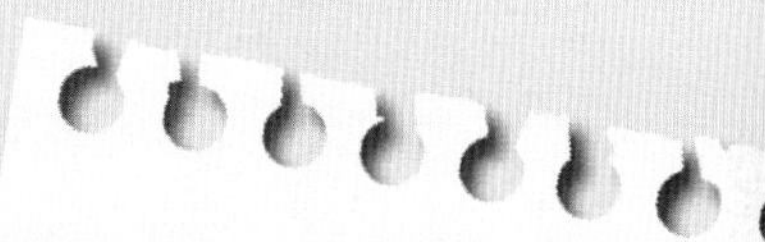

1. Visit several salons in your area (perhaps four or five). At each salon look at the way the staff present themselves, e.g. the way they dress, their hair and make-up, and so on.
2. Write a report on each of the salons about the way the staff looked (hair, make-up, clothing, etc.). Now you will need to decide whether you think the way the staff were presented was decided by the type of salon they were working in. Add these notes into your report.

Daily personal hygiene routine

It is important that you look after your personal hygiene when working in a salon. You will be working quite close to your clients so if you have body odour, it will be very unpleasant for them. To make sure you smell sweet every day it is important that you have a daily cleansing routine.

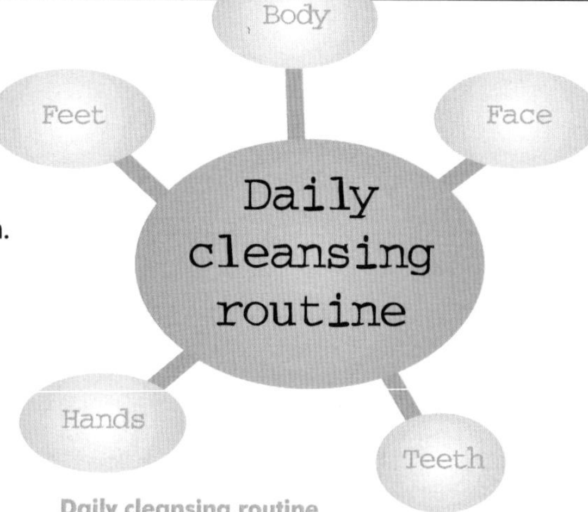

Daily cleansing routine

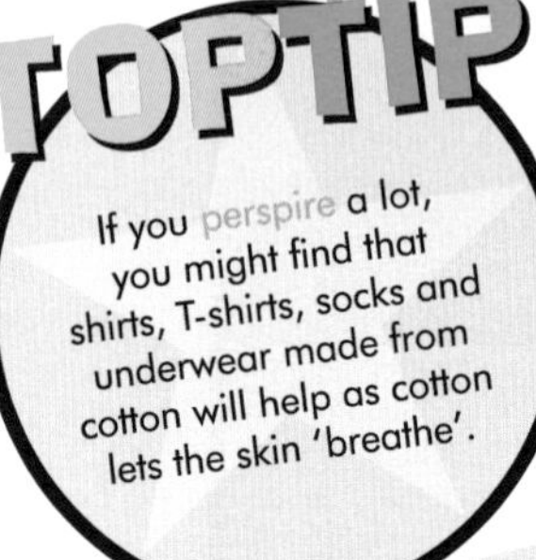

If you perspire a lot, you might find that shirts, T-shirts, socks and underwear made from cotton will help as cotton lets the skin 'breathe'.

sweat

The best way to keep clean is to bathe or shower every day using a mild soap or body wash and warm water. Wearing clean clothes, socks and underwear each day also helps you keep clean. Use a deodorant with antiperspirant so that you stay fresh. Talcum powder and foot sprays can also help lessen the odour of perspiring feet.

Daily cleansing of your face, teeth, hands and feet is also important. This will be covered in the next section.

Dear Nat

I work in a beauty salon and I love doing facial treatments on the clients, but I seem to perspire all the time. There are always wet marks under my arms, so I am embarrassed every time I have to lift up my arms or lean over a client. I don't know what to do about this. I've tried deodorants but nothing is helping. Please, please help. This problem is making me really miserable!

From Naomi

Nat says

Lots of people have problems with body perspiration. We all perspire different amounts and the odour of the sweat can be different from person to person. Some fabrics can make you perspire more than others, so have a look and see what your salon outfit is made from. Try and wear pure cotton clothes as these will help. You must make sure you get rid of the sweat, so bathe or shower at least once a day. You say you have tried lots of deodorants and they haven't worked. Perhaps try one with an antiperspirant in it – this will help to stop you perspiring and keep you dry.

Ways to ensure a good personal appearance

You will need to take care of your appearance. This is because you are your own best advertisement! If you look really well presented, it shows that you care about how you look and clients will think that you will do the same for them. Looking after your personal appearance includes:

- Face and skin care.
- Oral hygiene (taking care of your teeth).
- Nail care.
- Choosing the right clothing and keeping it looking good.
- Hair care.
- Hand care.
- Foot care.

Face and skin care

Keeping your face clean will not only make you look good but will also reduce the chance of spots. Do you know what your skin type is?

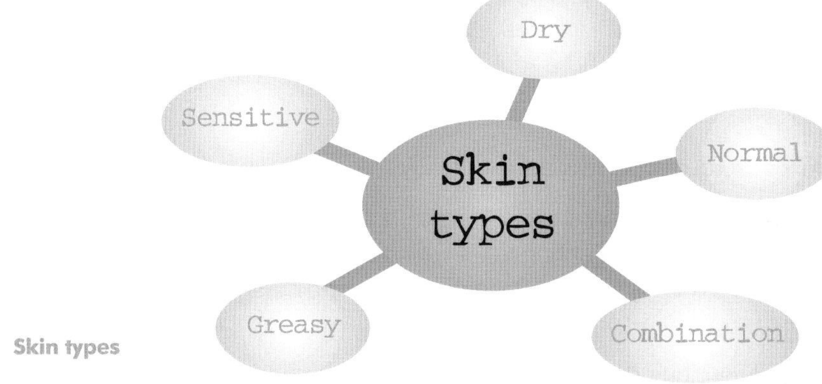

Skin types

TOP TIP

If you are not sure what type of skin you have, most department stores have make-up/skin care specialists who will be able to help you find out.

Whatever your skin type, you need to follow a good cleansing routine that should include:

- Cleansing.
- Toning.
- Moisturising.

Check that the products you use are the right ones for your skin type.

Your skin will show whether your diet and lifestyle are good or bad. If you eat lots of fatty foods such as chips, don't exercise or get enough sleep, your skin will start to show it!

If you wear make-up, you will need to make sure that it is appropriate for your working environment. Make-up should be subtle and applied correctly as this will make sure it looks good. Choose make-up products that are suitable for your skin type and which will enhance your face shape. Always remove make-up before you go to bed, otherwise it will block your pores and may cause spots. For information on how to apply make-up, see Unit 7 Basic make-up, page 132.

subtle: not very obvious

enhance: make more attractive

clear

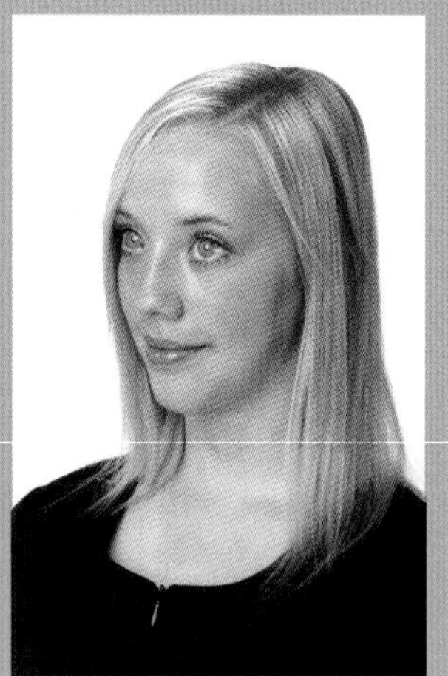

Appropriate make-up for a hair stylist or beauty therapist

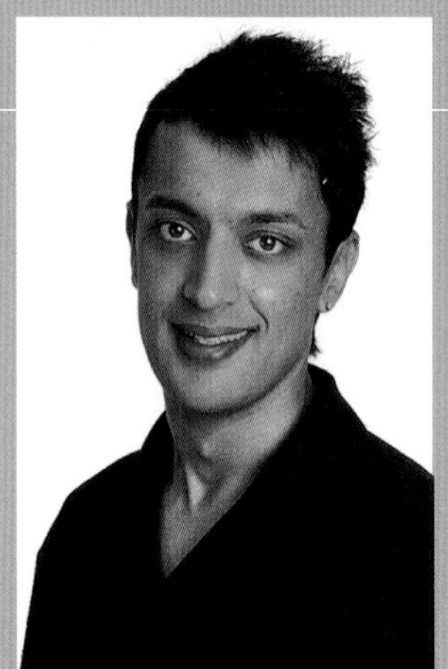

A well-presented male hairdresser

Some people choose not to wear make-up, which is great if you have a flawless, healthy skin that will look good without it. If your facial skin is greasy or you have spots, applying make-up over the top may make it worse. Most females look better wearing some make-up, even if it's just mascara and lip gloss. Beauty therapists often wear make-up because since they are selling make-up products to clients, it's a good selling point to wear it themselves!

Male hair stylists and therapists also need to make sure they are well presented. The face must be kept clean – the same cleanse, tone and moisturise routine may be followed. As well as having a clean face, men should ensure that facial hair is appropriate for the working environment. You could have:

- a clean shaven face
- a neat and well trimmed beard or
- well-presented 'designer stubble'.

Hair care

At work, it's important that your hair looks clean and tidy.

In the beauty salon, if your hair is below shoulder length, it should be tied up so it does not fall across the client you are working on. If your hair is short, it should be well styled and kept in good condition. You may need to wear hair slides or grips to stop your hair from falling over your face.

In the hairdressing salon your hair should make a statement. It should say 'Look at my hair, it's fabulous! You too could look as good as me'. The style of your hair and type of colouring techniques used will probably depend on how confident you are and the kind of salon you work in.

Below are some tips for keeping your hair looking shiny and healthy:

- Use the correct shampoo for your hair type. If your hair is colour treated, you should be using a shampoo and conditioner for colour-treated hair. If your hair is dry, use conditioner as this will help the hair to stay looking smooth and shiny.
- Have your hair trimmed regularly to avoid split ends and to keep your style looking good.
- If your hair needs to be tied up, make sure you use professional bands. Don't use ordinary elastic bands as these can damage the hair.
- Once you have shampooed (and conditioned your hair), treat it gently. Use a wide-tooth comb to remove any knots while the hair is wet. Start to comb the hair at the ends, then work up to the roots.
- Brush and comb your hair regularly to keep it looking tidy.

Oral hygiene

Oral hygiene is important in the salon as bad breath may cause offence to clients. You should clean your teeth with toothpaste at least twice a day and always before you go to bed. It is important to visit the dentist regularly to have your teeth checked (and treated if necessary). Untreated teeth can lead to bad breath.

to do with the mouth

Spicy foods and cigarettes can leave breath smelling unpleasant. Breath fresheners can be used to prevent this.

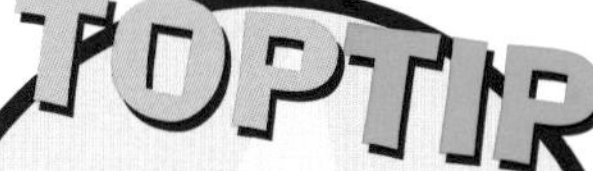

Use dental floss before brushing your teeth, as this will help to remove bits of food. Use a mouthwash after brushing to help stop plaque building up on your teeth. It will also make your mouth feel really clean and fresh!

Hand care

It is important to wash your hands regularly. If you are a beauty therapist, this should be done before you start each client. It is a good idea to use hand cream regularly to soften and protect your skin and prevent it from becoming dry, rough and chapped, especially in the cold weather.

You should always wash your hands before and after you have eaten, after you have sneezed and when you have used the toilet, as this will prevent germs spreading. Then dry your hands thoroughly, especially between your fingers. This will help to prevent contact dermatitis.

a skin condition that may be caused by regular contact with products such as shampoos and chemicals

Cover cuts or abrasions with a waterproof plaster to prevent cross infection

scrapes

infection being passed from one person to another

salon scene

Kat had started working in the hairdressing salon straight after leaving school, nearly six months ago. It was now the run up to Christmas and the salon was very busy. Kat seemed to spend most of her day at the basin, shampooing clients' hair. She was happy to do this because the atmosphere in the salon was a really happy one.

A few days before Christmas, Kat's finger started to itch really badly underneath the ring on her finger. The ring had belonged to Kat's gran, so it was very special to her and she liked to wear it all the time. At night time, the itching was dreadful. When she finished work on Christmas Eve, Kat took off the ring and was horrified to see her finger was bright red and was sore to the touch.

What do you think is wrong with Kat's finger?

What should she do now to try and help it to heal?

Nail care

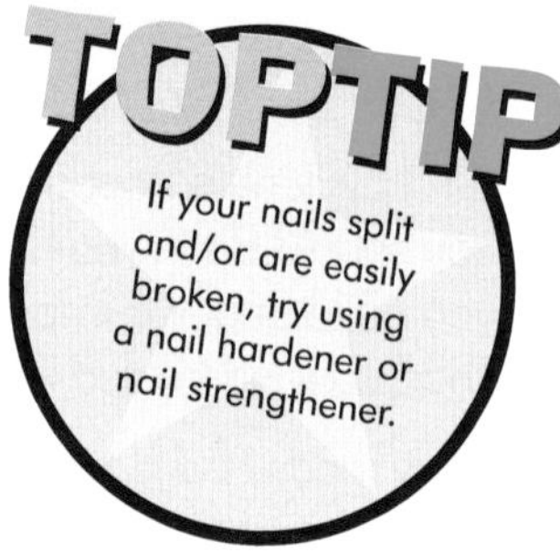

TOPTIP
If your nails split and/or are easily broken, try using a nail hardener or nail strengthener.

Finger nails should always be clean and kept fairly short, especially if you are a beauty therapist, as dirt and germs build up under long nails. Long nails may also scratch the client's skin, causing discomfort to the client. Some beauty clients have been known to have a reaction to the nail polish on the therapist's nails (your hands will be in contact with the client's skin). It is therefore best not to wear any nail polish. However, it is usually acceptable to wear nail polish if you are giving manicures or pedicures.

TOPTIP

Bitten nails look untidy, but there are products to help you stop biting your nails. These usually taste unpleasant so you won't want to bite your nails, but they are not poisonous!

Although nails without polish look cleaner and fresher, hair stylists may wear nail polish as long as it is unchipped and well presented. For information on how to apply and remove nail polish, see Unit 8 Basic manicure, page 154.

When shaping your nails it is best to cut them straight across and file off the sharp corners. When filing, always work from the outside of the nail in towards the middle. Use the file at a 45-degree angle to the nail. For more information on how to file nails, see Unit 8 Basic manicure, page 154.

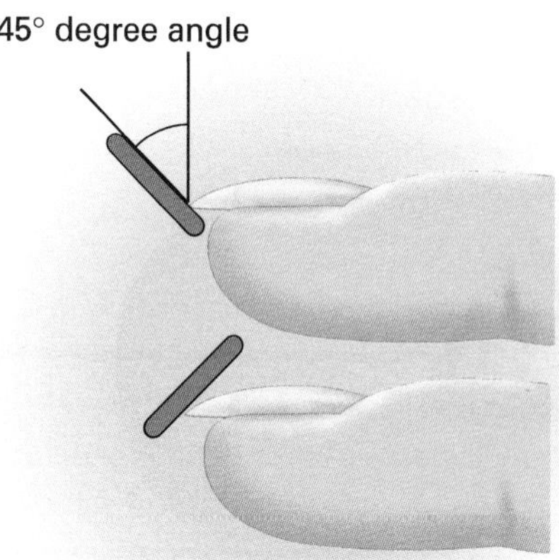

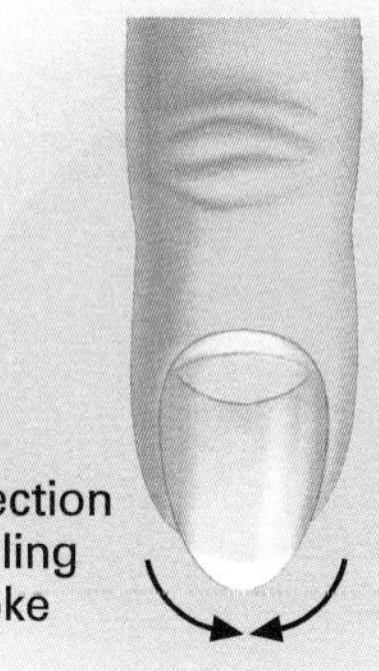

The right way to file nails

Foot care

During your daily bath or shower routine, remember to wash your feet and dry them thoroughly, especially between the toes. A pumice stone will help to remove hard skin on the soles of the feet, and foot creams will keep the skin soft and supple. If your feet perspire a lot during the day, foot sprays should help to prevent the odour.

pumice stone: a special stone for removing hard skin

supple: moveable, not stiff

Sometimes you may get problems with your feet, such as athlete's foot, corns or veruccas. These should be treated straightaway before they get really bad and cause you discomfort. The chemist will be able to advise you on a suitable treatment, or you may need to visit a chiropodist.

Long toenails may press against the end of your shoes and cause ingrowing toenails. The sides of your toes may become inflamed and sore to touch. Visit your doctor or a chiropodist if you have any pain or discomfort from ingrowing toe nails.

inflamed: the skin may go red or get hot

Choosing the right shoes

Sometimes fashion shoes look great but are not always good for your feet. Some shoes may change the shape of your feet and cause painful problems.

Since you will be spending a lot of time standing up when working in the salon, it is important to choose shoes that fit properly and meet certain health and safety requirements. Most good shoe shops will measure your feet to make sure the shoes you buy are the right fit. If your shoes don't fit properly, your legs and feet will ache by the end of the day.

Choose full shoes with closed-in toes and low heels. Shoes should be made of leather, as this allows the feet to breathe and will prevent unpleasant foot odour.

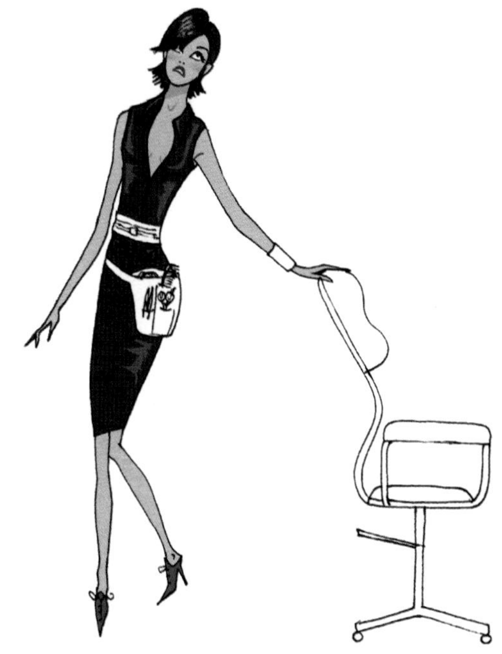

Wearing uncomfortable shoes will make your feet and legs ache by the end of the day

> Full, closed-in shoes are worn in the salon for health and safety reasons. They should protect your feet if you drop something sharp onto them. In the hairdressing salon, it will also stop tiny hairs from becoming stuck in the soles of your feet!

Choosing the right clothing

The clothing you wear in the salon should reflect the environment in which you are working.

What to wear in the beauty therapy salon

Beauty therapists should wear an appropriate salon dress or tunic because:

- it is hygienic (and helps to prevent cross infection)
- it presents a professional image
- it shows the salon's image
- it saves your own clothes from getting dirty.

The style of your salon dress or tunic will most probably be decided by the salon or your tutor. You will need to check that you have plenty of room to move your arms about while you are working.

What to wear in the hairdressing salon

The hairdressing salon tends to be less formal, as hairdressing is a fashion industry, and the clothing you wear should reflect this.

Your clothing must be appropriate for the salon. For example, if your top has flowing or loose baggy sleeves, these might get caught in electrical equipment. Imagine if your clothing were to get caught in the fan in the hairdryer. This would be dangerous.

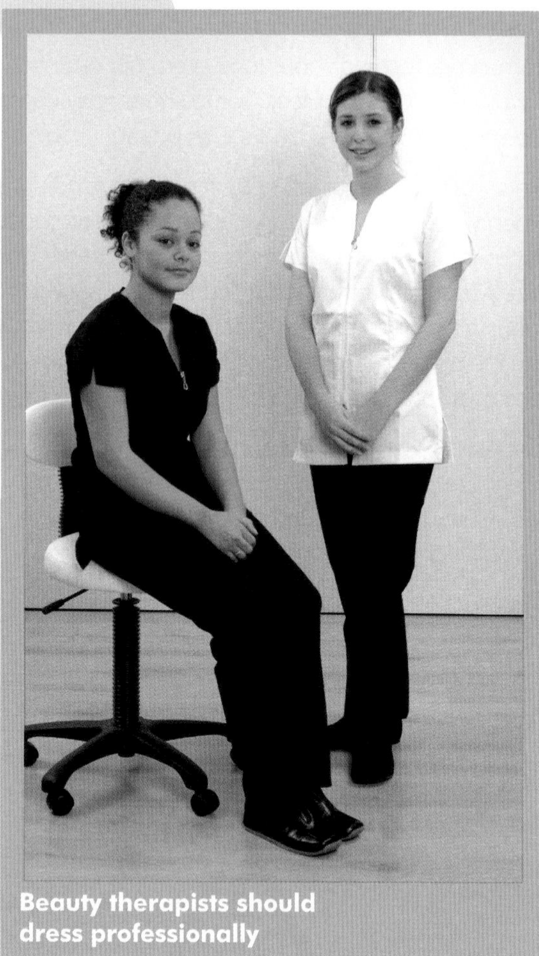

Beauty therapists should dress professionally

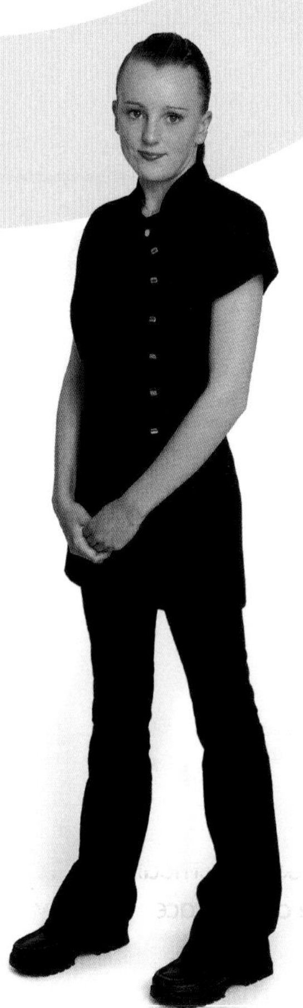

A well-presented hair stylist

You must also make sure you have room to stretch your arms, as you will need to be able to stretch and move your upper body when blow-drying, setting and so on.

Try to wear clothes that are made from cotton, as this fabric allows the skin to breathe. Also any hair cuttings can be easily brushed off cotton clothes. Hair can get caught in other fabrics such as woollen jumpers.

If your salon has a uniform, this should be worn as it makes sure everyone looks the same and also stops your own clothes from getting spoilt.

Dear Nat

I work in a fashionable salon where the stylists do really up-to-date work. Our boss keeps going on about 'hairdressing is a fashion industry', so why did he get so angry when I came into work wearing a crop top? I thought I looked really good and trendy, and so did the other staff.

From Zahra

Nat says

This is a tough one, as I can see both points of view. Yes, you are right, you should look fashionable, but your boss is also right as tops that show your stomach and arm-pits are not really appropriate for the salon. Showing your stomach doesn't look professional and imagine how your clients feel when you are shampooing their hair and they look up into your armpit! I'm sure you must have other fashionable tops in your wardrobe that don't show your stomach or armpits and I bet your boss would be really pleased if you wore one of them to work.

Wearing personal protective equipment

Sometimes your employer or tutor will tell you that it is necessary to wear personal protective clothing.

As a hair stylist, this would be gloves (to protect your hands from chemicals) and an apron (to protect your clothing or uniform from chemicals that might spill on to them).

As a beauty therapist, you may also be asked to wear gloves to protect your hands when using chemicals (cleaning products) for cleaning equipment. An apron can protect your uniform from getting dirty if you are assisting another therapist in a waxing treatment.

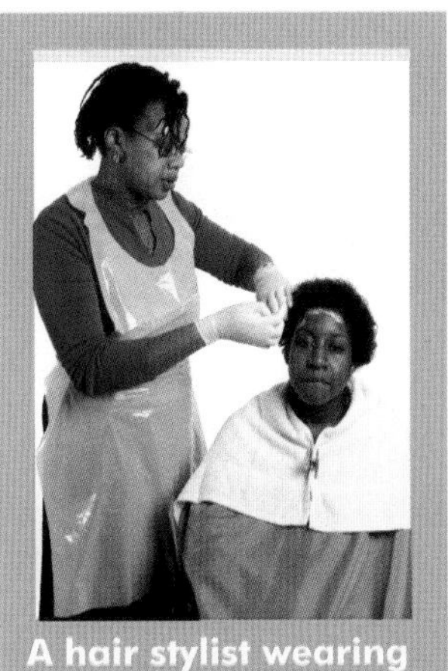

A hair stylist wearing protective clothing

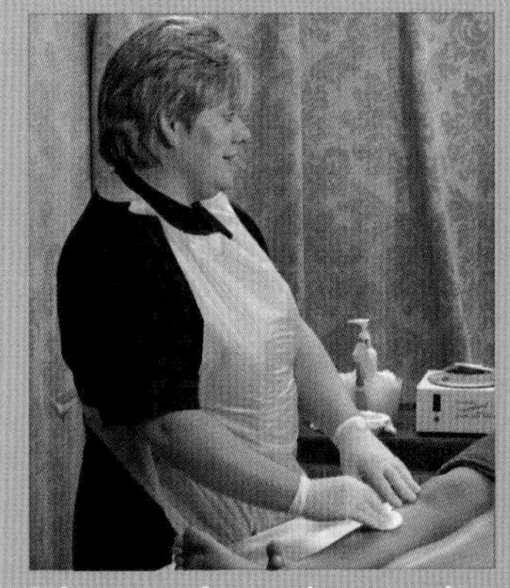

A beauty therapist wearing protective clothing

Jewellery

Any jewellery that you wear should be kept to a minimum. Health and safety problems may be caused if you are wearing lots of jewellery.

Beauty therapists should only wear a wedding ring and small stud earrings. This is because rings might scratch the client. Also, products can collect underneath them and cause dermatitis. Don't wear a watch as this could scratch the client's face and may increase the risk of cross infection.

Hair stylists should not wear rings for the same reasons as beauty therapists. Avoid long, dangly necklaces as these might get caught in equipment.

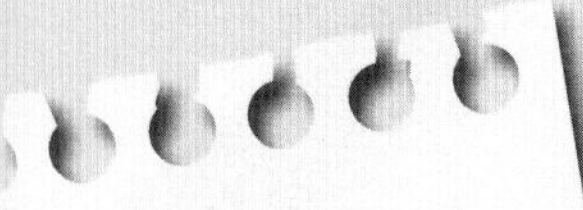

OVER TO YOU...

For this activity you will need to ask a number of people (e.g. family, friends) about their experiences of visiting a salon. You will need to find out the following:

1. What did they think about the way the staff presented themselves in the salon?
2. Did they feel more or less comfortable in a salon where all the staff wore uniforms?
3. Had they ever experienced a stylist or therapist with poor personal hygiene and, if they had, how did it make them feel?
4. Would they feel happy having their hair done by a stylist with greasy, untidy hair?
5. Would they feel happy having a nail treatment done by a therapist with bitten, dirty finger nails?

There may be other things regarding the presentation of staff that they will tell you about. Remember you can use your own experiences too!

Now write a report on whether the way staff present themselves in the salon affects the way customers feel.

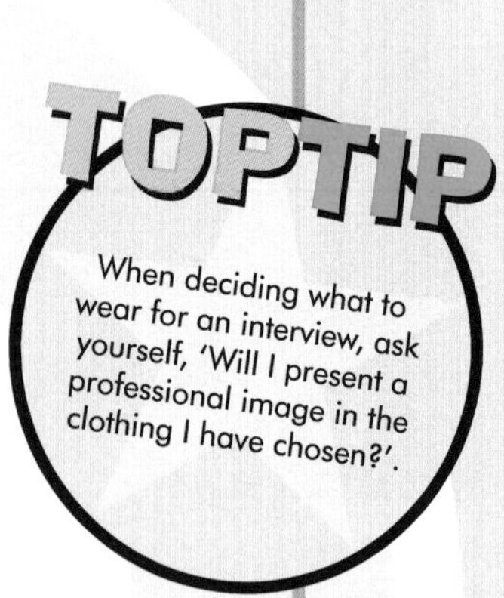

TOPTIP
When deciding what to wear for an interview, ask yourself, 'Will I present a professional image in the clothing I have chosen?'.

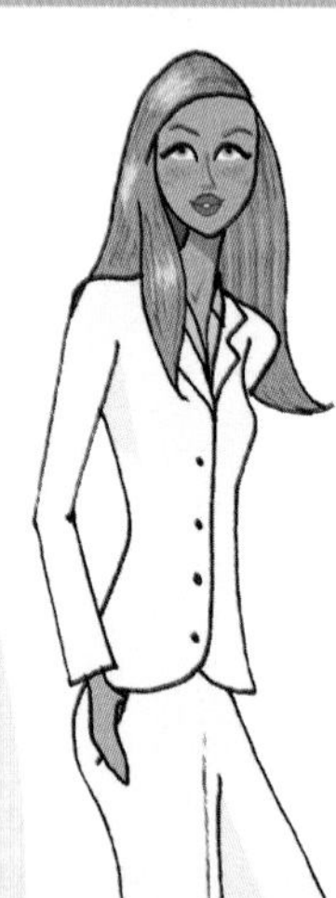

Knowing how to dress is important, but you must also look after the clothes you wear for work. They should be washed or dry cleaned regularly and ironed neatly. If they need mending, this should be done straightaway.

You will need to present a professional image at an interview

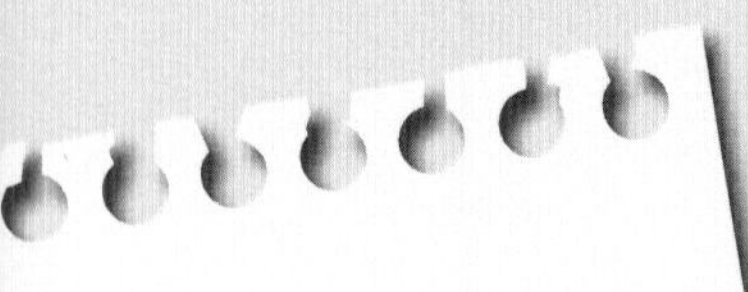

OVER TO YOU...

This activity should be done near the end of your course when you will have a good knowledge of this subject and possibly your own experiences to draw on. Earlier in the unit, you were asked to describe the kind of salon you would like to work in. Remember you must feel comfortable and happy in the salon. Have you changed your mind? Do you still feel the same way as you did at the beginning of the course? Give yourself some time to think about this and reflect on all the knowledge and experience you have gained.

Check what you know...

Watch out! Some questions have more than one correct answer.

1. Your clothing should always be in good condition when you are working in the salon because:
   - ☐ high fashion clothing is important
   - ☐ you must show a professional image at all times
   - ☐ you might be going out straight after work

2. If you find a verucca on your foot you should:
   - ☐ ignore it
   - ☐ see a doctor or buy some medication
   - ☐ take a bath

3. Nails should always be filed:
   - ☐ from the side to the centre
   - ☐ from the centre to the side
   - ☐ straight across

4. To remove bits of food before brushing your teeth:
   - ☐ use mouth wash
   - ☐ floss your teeth
   - ☐ eat an apple

5. A healthy meal consists of:
   - ☐ burger and chips
   - ☐ chicken, boiled potato, carrots, peas and fruit salad to follow
   - ☐ vegetable pizza with salad and chocolate fudge cake to follow

6. You shouldn't wear rings in the salon because:
   - ☐ your boss might not like them
   - ☐ someone might steal them
   - ☐ products can get underneath and cause dermatitis

7. Exercise is good for you because:
   - ☐ it makes you perspire
   - ☐ it can increase your energy levels
   - ☐ it makes your legs ache

8. To help prevent perspiration, the best material for clothes to be made from is:
   - ☐ wool
   - ☐ nylon
   - ☐ cotton

9. Closed-in shoes should be worn in the salon to:
   - ☐ make your feet perspire
   - ☐ please your boss
   - ☐ prevent you from injuring yourself if you drop something sharp on your feet

10. An antiperspirant should be used to:
    - ☐ make you smell fresh
    - ☐ remove sweat
    - ☐ stop or dry up sweat

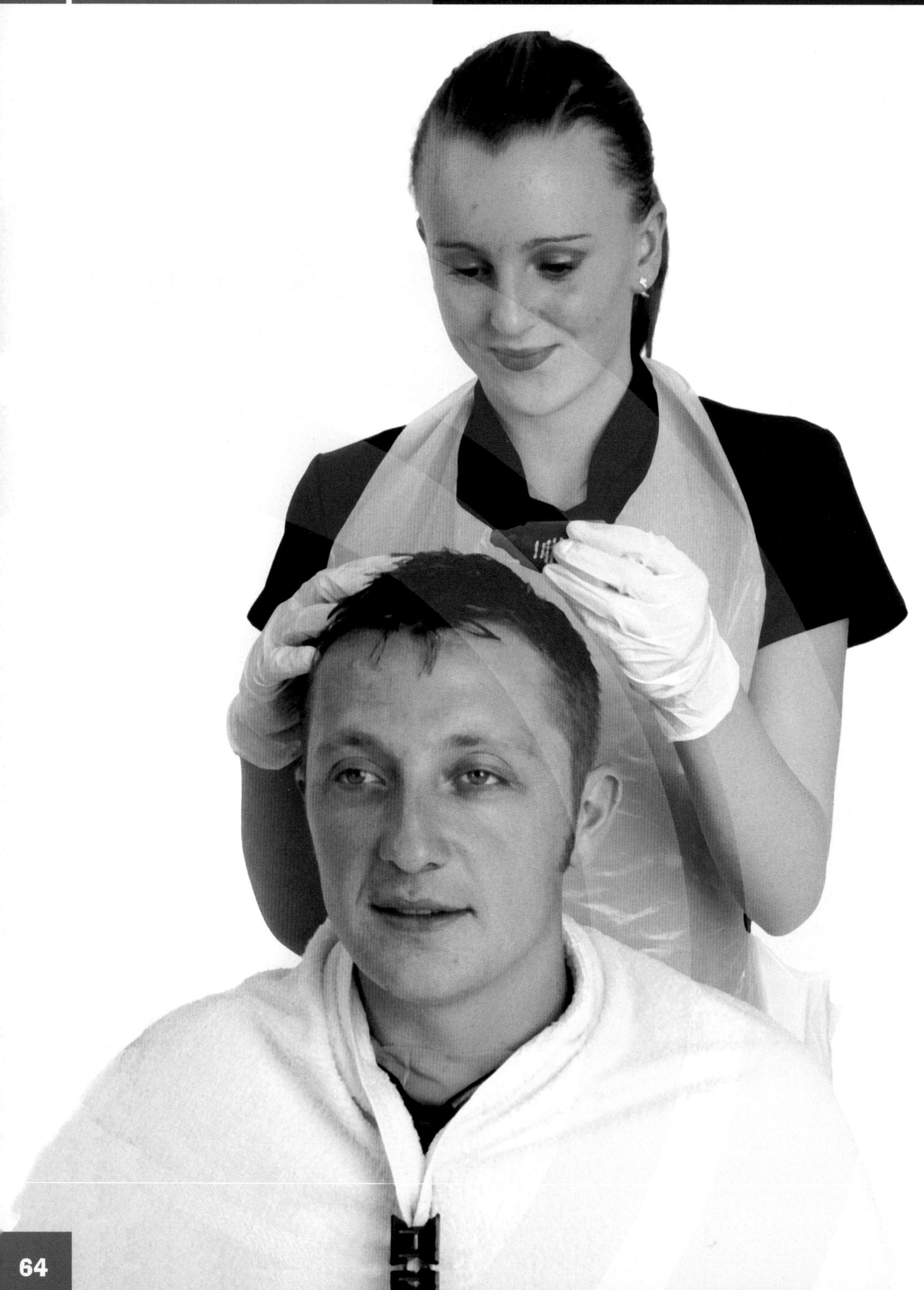

Unit 4

Health and safety

It is important that you work safely in the salon. This is to make sure that you, the people you work with and your clients are protected from harm. To work safely, you will have to follow certain rules and also look out for anything that could cause an accident. That way you will help to prevent accidents from happening, making the salon a safer place.

A lot of health and safety is basic commonsense, but sometimes you may feel it has nothing to do with you. However, as you read through this unit, you will see that it has a great deal to do with you!

In this unit you will learn about:

- Health and safety rules.
- Accidents and how to avoid them.
- Evacuating the salon in an emergency.

Towards the end of this unit, you will be observed and assessed on:

- Your safety consciousness.
- Safe working practice.

Health and safety rules

the people you work with

It is important that you follow health and safety rules in the salon. Your employer should tell you all about them. These rules are there to make sure you, your colleagues and clients stay free from harm.

Health and Safety at Work Act

This is the main health and safety law. (Most other health and safety laws are connected to the Health and Safety at Work Act.) When working in the salon you have responsibilities under the act and they are:

- To make sure you don't do anything that might put yourself or others in danger, e.g. running in the salon.
- To make sure you don't put yourself or other people in danger because you don't do something (or forget to do it). For example, if you notice water on the floor and you don't mop it up immediately, this may cause someone to slip and hurt themselves.
- To use anything that is given to you to help you to work safely in the correct way, e.g. gloves to prevent chemicals touching your hands.
- To report to your employer any accident or anything that might cause an accident in the salon, e.g. if you fall while you are at work. Your employer must record all accidents, no matter how small, in the salon's accident book.
- To help your employer carry out their health and safety responsibilities. For example, your employer has a duty to provide a fire exit so that people can leave the salon quickly if there is an emergency. If you notice that the fire exit is blocked by a pile of boxes, it is your duty to tell your employer – in an emergency a blocked fire exit could mean the difference between life and death.

follow

It isn't just you who has to comply with the health and safety rules. The law also states there are several things that your employer must do to ensure that employees, including you, and clients are kept safe and healthy. They include the following:

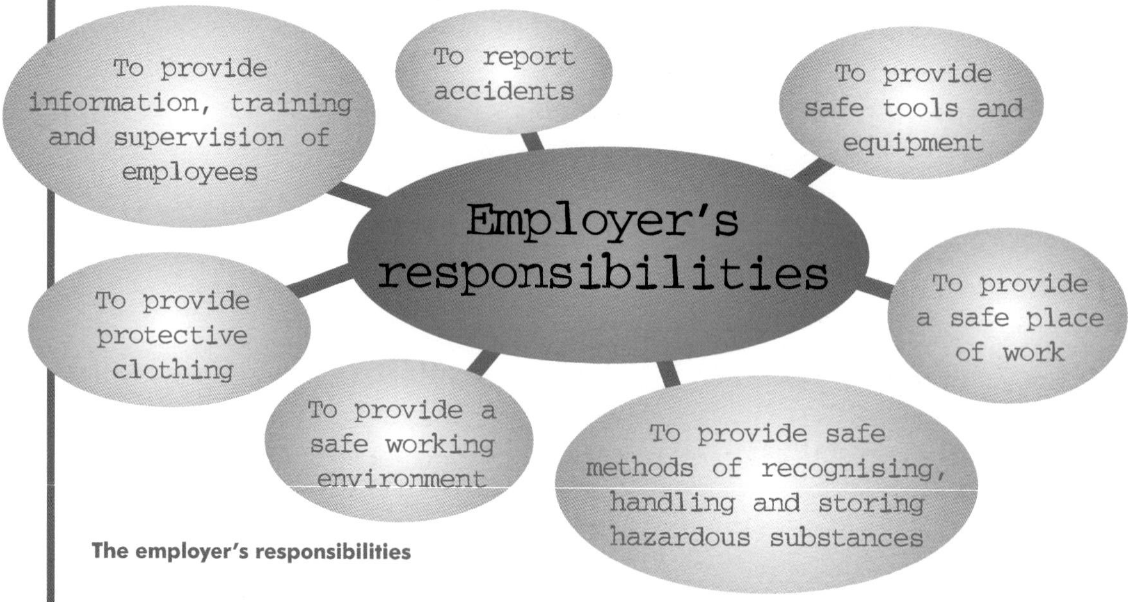

Employer's responsibilities

To provide information, training and supervision of employees

To report accidents

To provide safe tools and equipment

To provide a safe place of work

To provide safe methods of recognising, handling and storing hazardous substances

To provide a safe working environment

To provide protective clothing

The employer's responsibilities

The salon also has to have its own health and safety policy, which sets out the employer's rules and guidelines for ensuring all employees and clients are safe. You will need to follow these rules and guidelines. Your employer has to review the health and safety policy at regular intervals to make sure it is working well.

check

Hazards and risks

Throughout this unit, you will come across the terms 'hazard' and 'risk'. It is important that you understand what the difference is as this will help you to better understand health and safety.

A hazard is something that could possibly cause an accident or an injury, for example a spillage of water on the floor.

A risk is the chance that an accident might happen because of the hazard, for example someone slipping and falling on the wet floor.

A safe place of work

Your employer has to provide you with a safe place of work. The entrance to the salon and exits must allow clear and safe access. There should be no loose carpet or floor tiles, so you cannot trip over them and hurt yourself.

You should have enough space to work comfortably without bumping into work stations or other salon staff.

All fire exits must be clearly marked so, if there is a fire, everyone knows where to go. Your employer also has to make sure you know where the assembly point is, in case you have to leave the building in an emergency.

They should also make sure you have somewhere to keep your coat and bags etc.

Safe tools and equipment

Your employer has a responsibility to make sure any tools or equipment that you use in the salon are well constructed, maintained and safe to use.

put together

looked after

All electrical equipment should be tested at least once a year by a qualified electrician and your employer should keep records to prove this. You must make sure equipment stays safe to use in between the electrical tests. You can do this by:

- Making sure the flex (wire) is not frayed or split open before you use it, as this could cause someone to be injured.
- Removing from use any electrical equipment that is broken or faulty – tell your manager.
- Making sure hot items have cooled down before they are put away, e.g. wax pots, curling tongs.
- Checking plugs and plug sockets are not broken.

You should also only use equipment that you have been trained to use. This is to prevent you from injuring either yourself or someone else because you don't know what you are doing. For example, if used incorrectly, both a facial steamer and a hairdressing steamer could scald a client.

All hairdressing tools and non-electrical equipment should be checked before use. For example, combs should have all their teeth as broken teeth could scratch the client's scalp and cause cross infection. Beauty therapy tools and equipment should also be checked regularly to make sure they are in good working condition.

cross infection: infection being passed from one person to another

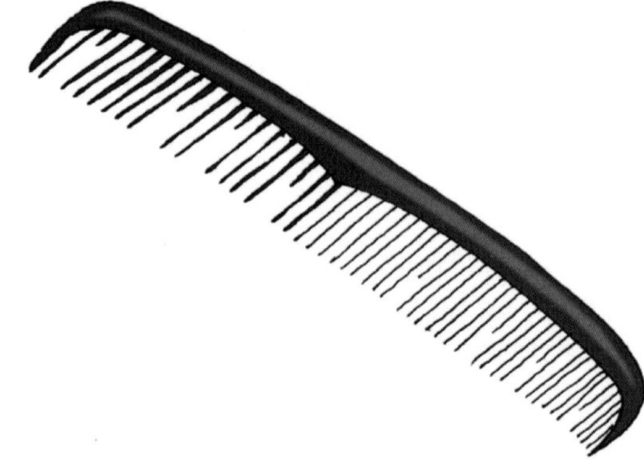

Never use damaged tools

Equipment should be placed on a sturdy surface to make sure nothing will fall off and cause an accident such as a chemical jar falling to the floor and breaking.

sturdy: strong and firm

salon scene

Flick had been working in the hairdressing salon on a Saturday for the past four months. The salon owner had been very good to her and had showed her how to shampoo, remove colours and neutralise perms. Apart from this, Flick made cups of tea and coffee for the clients and washed and dried all the towels.

One Saturday, one of the stylists had phoned in sick, so Flick found that she was extra busy. She was asked to get a climazone and put a client under it. She had seen the stylists do this – it was easy. You just wheeled the climazone over to the client, opened up the arms, put the client underneath and switched it on, so that was what she did. As the salon was busy, no one noticed that the client was not sitting directly in the middle; one side of her head was closer to the heated arms of the climazone than the other. When the climazone 'pinged', the stylist went over to check that the client's bleach packets were ready. Unfortunately, one side of the client's hair (the one that had been too close to the heat source) had over processed.

Was this Flick's fault, or the fault of the stylist who had asked her to put the client under the climazone?

Should Flick have been using electrical equipment that she had not been trained to use?

Sterilisation

Sterilisation is the complete destruction of germs or bacteria by heat or chemical means. It is essential that tools used in the salon are free from germs to ensure everyone is safe, so all tools must be sterilised before use. This is to prevent cross infection .

There are several different methods of sterilisation:

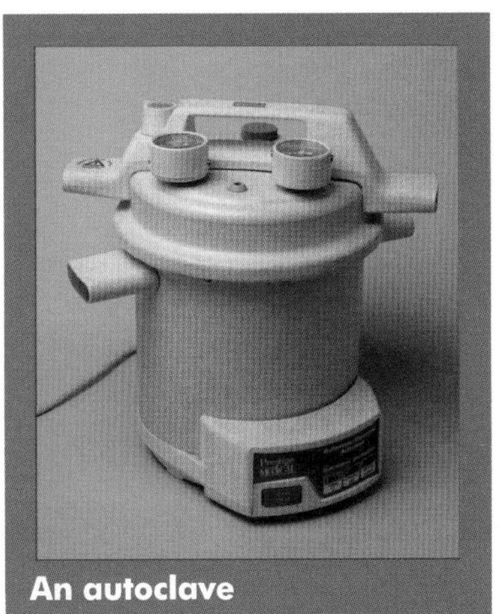

An autoclave

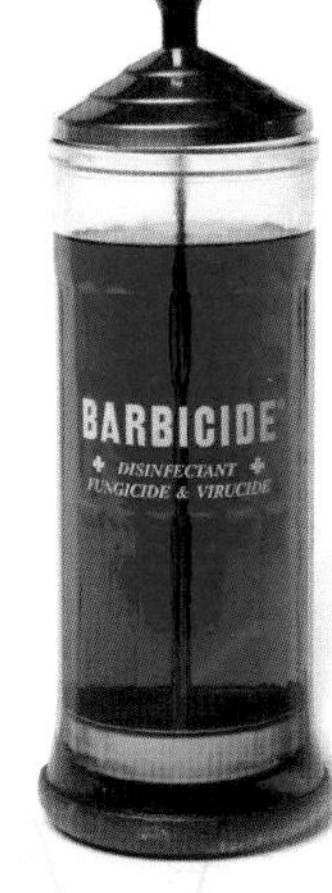

A chemical jar used in hairdressing salons

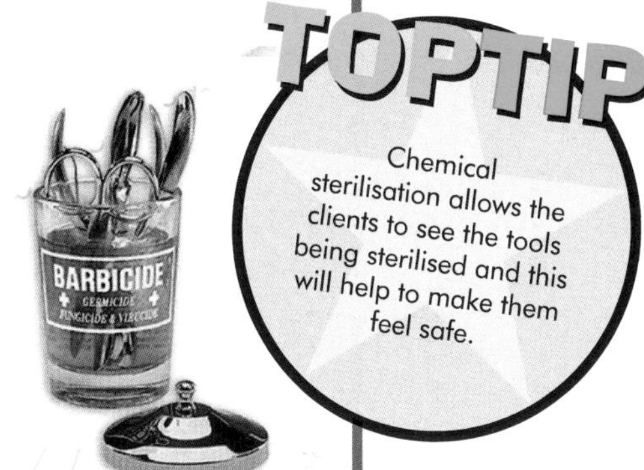

A small chemical jar used in beauty salons

TOP TIP

Chemical sterilisation allows the clients to see the tools being sterilised and this will help to make them feel safe.

- Steam sterilising (using an autoclave) – this is the best method for sterilising metal tools such as tweezers, scissors, etc. An autoclave works like a pressure cooker, so take care that it has cooled down thoroughly before removing your tools to avoid scalds or burns.
- Chemical sterilisation – this is used widely in both hairdressing and beauty salons. The chemical sterilising mixture should be made up following the manufacturer's instructions and used correctly – tools must be completely covered by the fluid and left in for the right length of time or else the tools will not be sterilised.

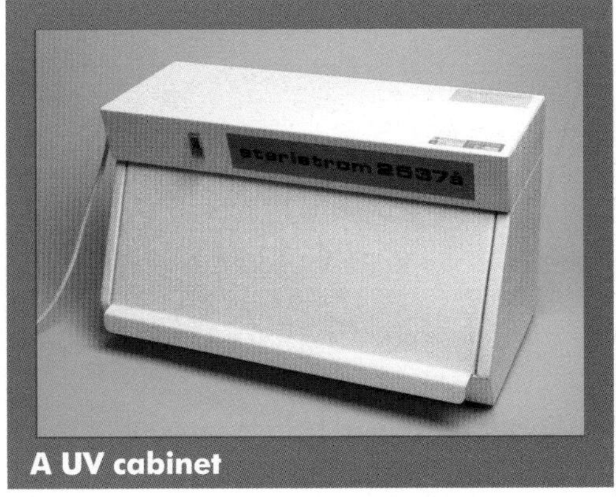

A UV cabinet

- Sterilisation using ultra-violet rays – this is also a popular method of sterilisation. The ultra-violet (UV) rays (like those on a sun bed) are used to sterilise tools and equipment. The UV rays come from the top of the cabinet and sterilise the surfaces that they hit. Therefore, you must make sure you turn tools over to ensure all parts are sterilised. Tools should be sterilised for 20 minutes on each side.

All tools should be washed/cleaned before you sterilise them.

Dear Nat

I am training to be a beauty therapist and really enjoy working with people and seeing them look good when they leave the salon. The one thing that really gets me down is all this cleaning and sterilising business. The other day I put one of the therapist's manicure tools into the sterilising fluid without washing them first. She was furious. I can't see what the problem is – they're going to be clean when they come out.

From Petra

Nat says

I can see where you're coming from, but the therapist is right. The manicure tools should have been cleaned before they went into the steriliser. If you put tools into the steriliser that haven't been cleaned first, the sterilisation won't be fully effective so germs can still spread.

I know a lot of beauty salons use disposable tools wherever possible, so the need for sterilising tools is less. However, if the tools are to be used again, it is really important that they are properly clean. How would you like it if someone else's skin or nail filings were on manicure tools that were used on your hands? The client before you could have had an infectious condition that would then be passed on to you. I hope this helps you to see how important correct sterilisation is.

Protective clothing

You may be required to wear protective clothing when you are carrying out certain services or when cleaning if you are using detergent, etc. Your employer will carry out a risk assessment to decide what the best kind of protective clothing for the job is and will then provide this for you.

Personal protective clothing includes the following:

- Gloves – these will protect your hands from chemicals and should help to prevent dermatitis. Beauty therapists may also wear gloves during the waxing service to prevent the risk of cross infection.
- Aprons – these are worn to protect your clothes/uniform from chemicals and spillages.

It is your responsibility to wear the protective clothing provided, if your employer says it is necessary for health and safety.

A safe working environment

Your employer has to provide you with a safe environment in which to work, as follows:

- The salon temperature should be comfortable to work in – between 18 – 21°C. It should also be warm enough for clients, particularly those who may need to undress for a beauty treatment or who have wet hair. However, the salon must not be so warm that it makes the stylist or therapist feel ill.
- There should be enough light for the stylist or therapist to work in. Poor lighting can strain your eyes.
- A good ventilation system will prevent the salon becoming humid. A humid atmosphere will make you feel tired more quickly and is an ideal environment for germs to spread. In the beauty salon, a ventilation system will remove fumes from nail polishes and acetone (used in nail polish remover), which can cause severe headaches and sickness.

humid: air feels damp, heavy and warm

- There may be a dust hazard from certain chemicals or processes (e.g. powder bleach used in the hairdressing salon). You might have to wear a face mask when working with these chemicals. Filing nails produces dust, which is something to consider if you suffer from any respiratory problems such as asthma. Dust and/or fumes may bring on an attack.

respiratory: breathing

- The salon should have a suitable staff toilet, washroom (with soap) and a way of drying your hands, e.g. paper towels. Special bins should be provided for you to dispose of sanitary items such as tampons.

Dealing with harmful substances

Most of the chemicals you will come into contact with in the salon can be harmful if they are used incorrectly. Your employer has a duty to ensure you are as safe as possible when working with these substances.

To help you work safely, your employer has to:

- Assess the risk to your health from using harmful substances and then decide the best way to keep you safe and healthy.

assess: work out

- Tell you about the risks involved and what precautions you must take, e.g. wearing protective clothing.
- Train you to work safely when handling chemicals.

You may be given the above information verbally and/or in writing.

Your employer will check to make sure that you are handling chemicals in the correct way. They will also fill in forms to confirm that your health is being monitored in relation to the use of harmful substances.

All substances that are harmful have an identification label on them. The different symbols will tell you the way in which they are harmful.

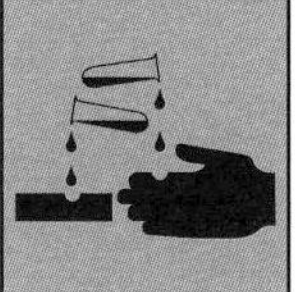
corrosive

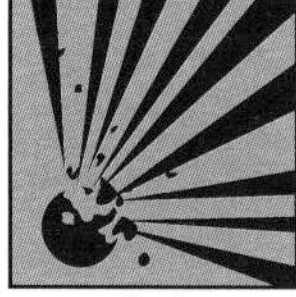
explosive

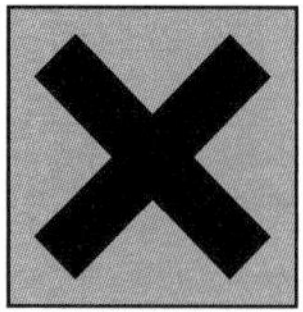
irritant

highly flammable

oxidizing

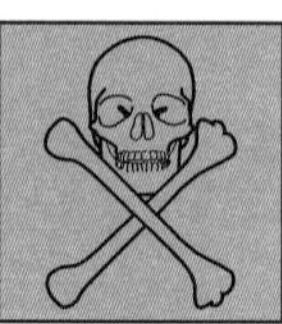
toxic

Symbols showing the different types of dangerous substances

There should be information in the salon regarding each chemical substance that you may have to work with.

> You may have seen the safety symbols above before in your science labs at school or at home on bottles containing cleaning products. To make sure you are as safe as possible, always read the manufacturer's instructions.

10A Hair Colorant – Semi-Permanent (Non-Aerosol)

Composition
Solutions of direct dyestuffs in a shampoo base which may be liquid, cream or gel.

Ingredients
Dyestuffs – up to 10%
Solvents (e.g. glycols or glycol ethers) – up to 10%
Ethanol – up to 50%

Hazards Identification
Refer to manufacturer's pack list of declarable dyestuffs which, if present, may require a sensitivity test before use.
May be flammable.

First Aid Measures
Eyes: Rinse eyes immediately with plenty of water. If irritation persists, seek medical advice.
Skin: Wash skin immediately (mainly to avoid staining).
Ingestion: Drink 2–3 glasses of water or milk. Seek medical advice immediately.

Accidental Release Measures
Use plenty of water to dilute and mop up spillages.

Fire-fighting Measures
Use carbon-dioxide or dry powder extinguisher.

Handling & Storage
Avoid contact with eyes and face. Do not use on abraded or sensitive skin. Store in a cool place away from direct sunlight and other sources of heat. Use away from sources of ignition.
Liquid products may contain alcohol which makes the product flammable; keep small quantities in the salon for immediate use only.

Exposure Controls/ Personal Protection
Apply in a well-ventilated area. Always wear suitable protective gloves.

Disposal
Do not incinerate. Wash down the drain with plenty of water.

Example of hazard data sheet giving information about a chemical substance used in the hairdressing salon

Nail polish remover

Composition
Liquid.

Ingredients
Ethyl acetate
Isopropyl alcohol
Water

Hazards Identification
Refer to manufacturer's instructions. May be flammable. Known irritant. Avoid inhalation.

First Aid Measures
Eyes: Flush out immediately with plenty of cold water. If irritation persists, seek medical advice.
Skin: Rinse immediately with cold water. If irritation persists, seek medical advice.

Accidental Release Measures
Absorb with tissue. Seal in a plastic bag for commercial waste disposal.

Fire-fighting Measures
Dry powder extinguisher.

Handling & Storage
Avoid contact with eyes and face. Do not use on abraded or sensitive skin. Store in a cool place away from direct sunlight and other sources of heat. Use away from sources of ignition.

Exposure Controls/ Personal Protection
Apply in a well ventilated area.

Disposal
Wash down the drain with plenty of cold water.

Example of hazard data sheet giving information about a chemical substance used in the beauty therapy salon

When dealing with chemicals you will also need to think about the following:

- How and where they are stored, e.g. aerosols should never be stored on a warm, sunny window ledge as the heat could cause them to explode. They should be stored away from heat and sunlight.
- The correct way to dispose of them:
  - Left-over colouring products should be rinsed down the sink with plenty of running water.
  - Waste from a manicure service such as used cotton wool with nail polish remover, nail polish and/or cuticle remover should be placed in a bin liner in a small bin. At the end of each service the bin liner should be removed from the bin and tied. This should then be placed into an industrial waste bin. The salon should have a contract with a special refuse collection company.

contract: agreement

Dear Nat

I love my job in the salon. I don't even mind all the cleaning at the end of the day! The other day we had some health and safety training about harmful chemicals that we use in the salon. I didn't know about any of this, but now I'm worried because I think I should be wearing rubber gloves and maybe even a face mask when I'm using cleaning products in the salon. When I mentioned this to the stylists, they just laughed at me. They said that when they were training they all cleaned without gloves and a mask and it didn't do them any harm. What should I do?

From Samia

Nat says

The government is concerned about the long-term effects of using harmful substances in salons. Your employer will have done a risk assessment of all the products used in the salon (this includes cleaning products) and introduced ways to keep you safe while using them.

When you did your health and safety training, if your employer said that you should be wearing gloves and a mask when cleaning, then you should. I know it's hard, but you must try and ignore the silly comments that are made by people at work. You must think about your own health and safety, even if they don't think about theirs. They aren't working within the rules of health and safety, as these rules state that you shouldn't do anything that might put yourself, your colleagues or your clients at risk. As you are one of their colleagues, they could be putting your health and safety at risk by the way they are behaving. Stay safe!

Reporting accidents

All accidents at work, no matter how small, must be reported in full and recorded in the accident book. There is usually one person responsible for completing the accident book, but the information regarding the accident may come from anyone who witnessed it. By keeping records your employer will be able to see if there is a problem and then put it right. If the accident is serious, it must be reported to the Health and Safety Executive.

government organisation responsible for looking into health and safety at work

ACCIDENT REPORT FORM

This form must be completed in all cases of accident, injury or dangerous occurrence.

Name of person reporting the accident	Activity at time of injury/accident
Position in organisation	Place of injury/accident
Name of injured person	First aid treatment given (if any)
Date of birth	Was the injured person taken to hospital? If so, where?
Position in organisation	Name(s) and position(s) of person(s) present when the accident occured
Date and time of accident	Details of injury/accident
Signature of person reporting accident and date Signature Date	

An accident report form

TRY IT OUT!

Find out where the accident report book is kept in your salon.

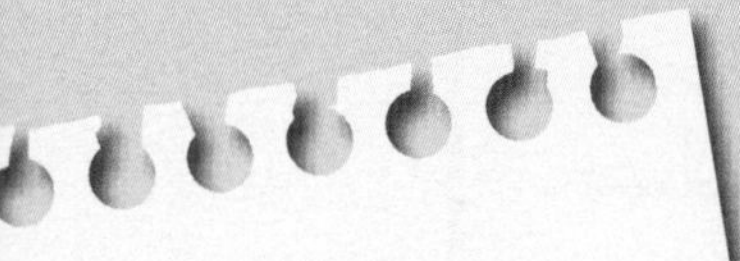

OVER TO YOU...

Describe what responsibilities your employer has for health and safety in the workplace under the Health and Safety Act. What are your own responsibilities as an employee under the Health and Safety Act? What other duties do you have when working in a salon to keep it a healthy and safe place to work?

Accidents and how to avoid them

Accidents will happen no matter how careful you are, but while you are in the salon you need to act professionally, watch out for anything that could cause an accident and then deal with the situation to prevent the accident from happening. You will need to think about the health and safety training you have been given and decide, for example, whether you should be wearing protective clothing. If in doubt, ask a senior member of staff.

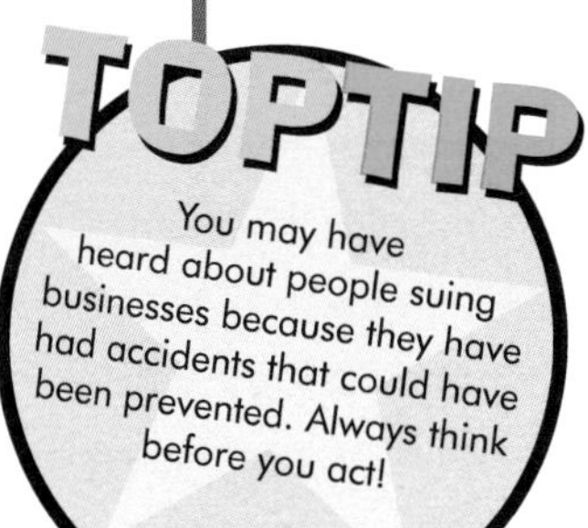

TOPTIP
You may have heard about people suing businesses because they have had accidents that could have been prevented. Always think before you act!

Most accidents in the salon happen as a result of someone doing something that is unsafe or because the workplace is unsafe. Often human error will be involved, for example poor health and safety training, carelessness or unprofessional behaviour. Accidents are usually caused by human factors or environmental factors – some examples are given in the tables below.

Examples of accidents caused by human factors

Human factors	Example	What may happen
Carelessness	Ignoring trailing wires Not wiping up a spillage	Someone may trip Someone may slip
Inappropriate behaviour	Running around the salon Spraying water at someone	You may slip and fall, especially if there is water on the floor (from the water spray)
Inappropriate dress	Tops with long floaty sleeves	A sleeve may fall onto the client's face or get caught in electrical equipment, e.g. a hairdryer
Tiredness	Too many late nights	You may become clumsy and knock things over. You may forget to do something, e.g. move boxes blocking a fire exit
Alcohol and drug taking	Drinking and drug taking can cause poor concentration, tiredness and poor coordination	You are likely to make a mistake, become clumsy and give a poor service

Examples of accidents caused by environmental factors

Environmental factors	Example	What may happen
Faulty tools and equipment	Frayed flexes on electrical equipment, e.g. hairdryers or wax pots	You could be electrocuted.
Chemicals stored incorrectly	Heavy or glass bottles stored on a high shelf	If you stretch up to reach the bottles and they fall, you could be injured.
Untidy and dirty work areas	Work area left dirty and untidy after a manicure or hair colouring service	Someone may knock something over, e.g. a chemical jar. Dirty work areas will put clients off returning to your salon and may also cause cross infection.
Poor salon layout	Work areas with sharp edges	Someone may walk into them and hurt themselves.

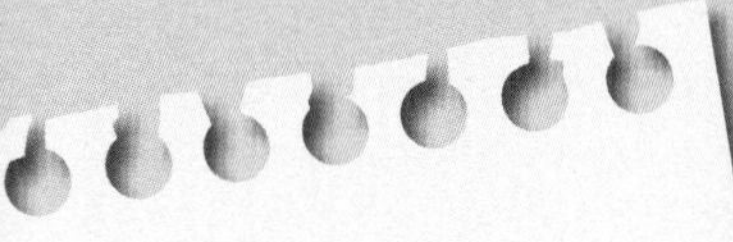

OVER TO YOU...

Look around the salon where you work and see if you can spot any hazards (e.g. physical hazards such as boxes, and hazards relating to fire, chemical storage and electrical equipment). Think carefully about what might happen if you ignore the hazards. Note down your answers and then decide what you should do about each one. An example is shown in the table below.

Check your answers with your tutor.

Hazard	What might happen?	What should I do?
A broken mirror	Someone could cut themselves	Report it to the salon manager so the bits of glass can be put into a **sharps bin**.

sharps bin: a special bin for putting glass and sharp objects such as razor blades

First Aid

All salons must have a first aid box. There should be someone who is responsible for ensuring it contains the right items and is kept fully stocked.

Salons should also have a member of staff responsible for first aid, although this person does not need to be a first aider (unless the salon employs over a certain number of people). He or she is responsible for deciding whether to send staff home if they are ill, call an ambulance if there is accident in the salon and so on.

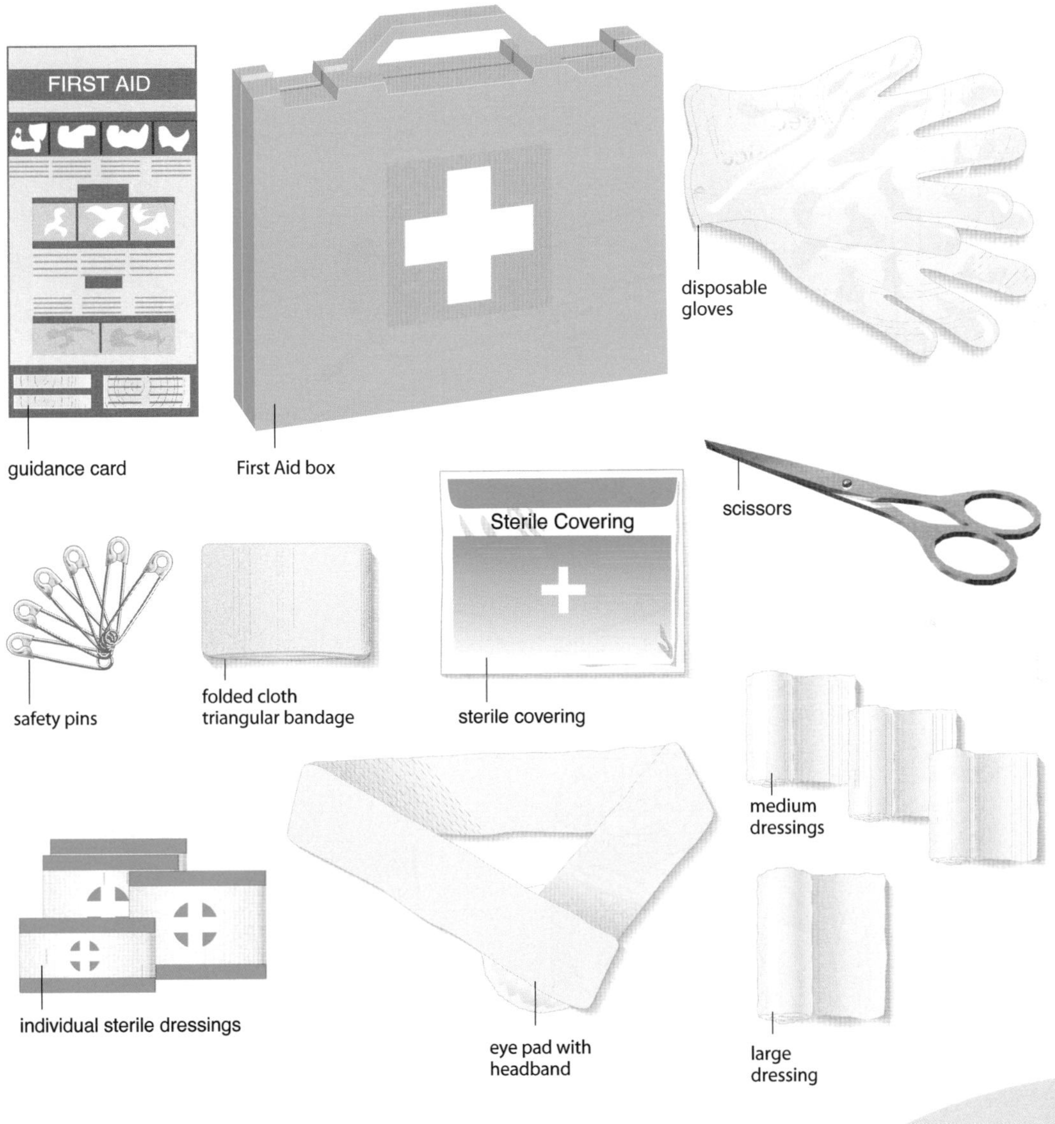

The contents of a first aid box

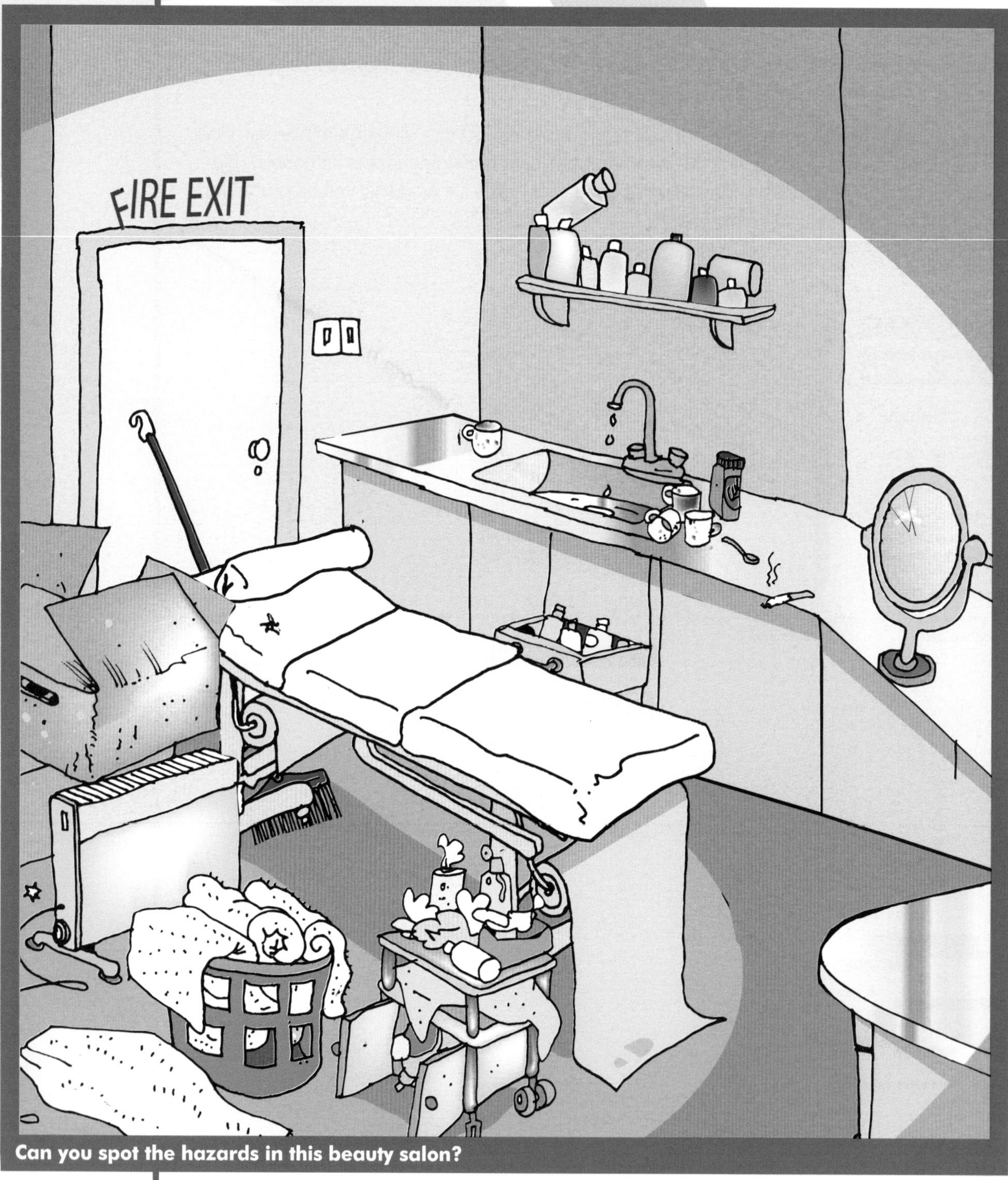

Can you spot the hazards in this beauty salon?

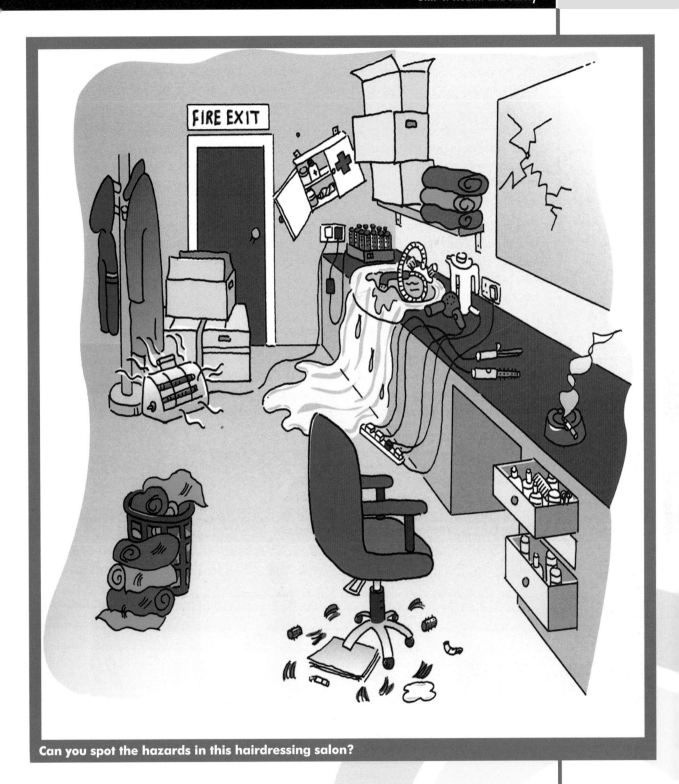

Can you spot the hazards in this hairdressing salon?

Your posture

The way you sit or stand – your posture – in the salon is important. If you sit or stand incorrectly, you may injure yourself. It also makes it more difficult to carry out the service on your client and you will quickly feel tired.

Sometimes it is not obvious that you have poor posture, but in the evening you may notice your neck and shoulders start to ache and feel stiff. This is because you have been working in an awkward position and have strained some muscles. In the long term, if you do not correct your posture now, you may find you have severe back pain as you get older.

very bad

When standing, your back should be straight, with your feet slightly apart and your weight evenly distributed (i.e. don't stand with all your weight on one leg) . If you need to bend, always bend your knees instead of your back. This may feel uncomfortable at first, but you will get used to it. When sitting, your back should be straight against the back of the chair, with your feet on the floor.

Lifting objects safely

When you lift a heavy object such as your school bag or a box of stock, do you ever stop to think about the way you are lifting it? The chances are if you need to pick something up from the floor, you bend your back. If the object is heavy, you can injure yourself lifting in this way.

TOP TIP

If you know a box is going to be difficult to lift or carry, either use a trolley to move it or ask someone to help you.

It is difficult to work in the salon if your back hurts, so try following these simple rules for lifting large or heavy objects:

1. Bend your knees and not your back.
2. Use both hands to hold the box.
3. Use your leg muscles to help you to stand up.

Think about the lift. Where is the load to be placed? Do you need help?

Get ready to lift. Stand with your feet apart.

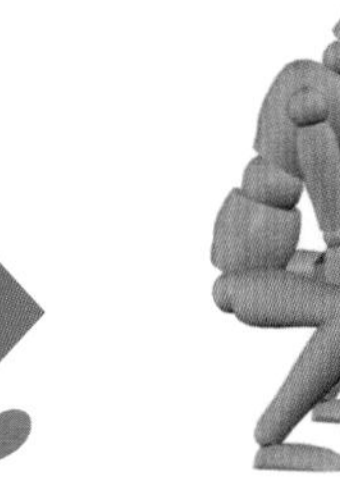

Bend your knees. Keep your back straight. Tuck in your chin. Lean slightly forward over the load to get a good grip.

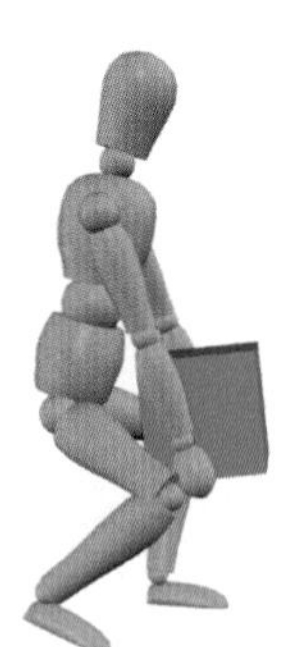

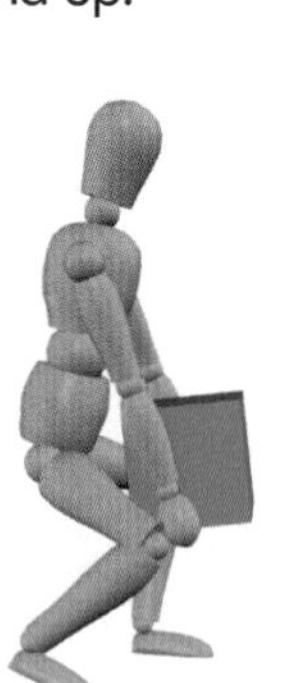

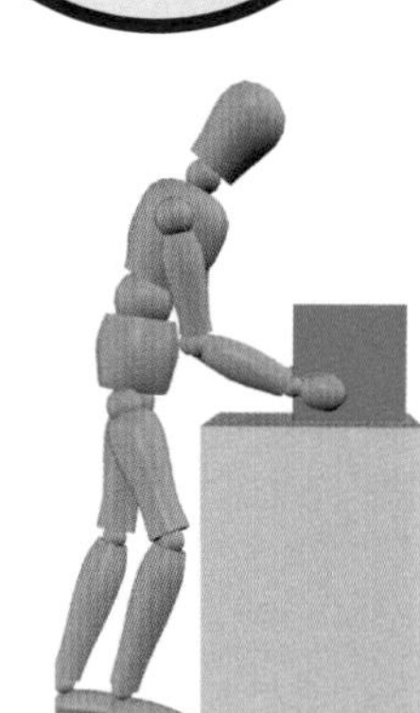

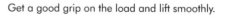

Get a good grip on the load and lift smoothly.

How to lift large objects

If you need to lift a large or heavy object from a shelf, make sure you use a sturdy step ladder and hold the object firmly, keeping it close to your body before you climb down the steps. You can also ask one of your colleagues to hold the step ladder to make sure it does not move.

The importance of good health and hygiene

To remind you how to maintain good health and hygiene, look back at Unit 3 Personal presentation, page 46.

Below are some likely hazards relating to poor health and hygiene.

The results of poor hygiene

Hazard	What might happen?	What should I do?
Going to work if you have an infectious or contagious condition such as a heavy cold	You might pass your germs to other members of staff and clients.	Report it to your employer.
Not washing your hands after using the toilet	You could pass germs on to other people.	Make sure you always wash your hands after using the toilet.
Long finger nails	You might scratch and injure the client.	Keep your nails short.

Evacuating the salon in an emergency

There may be times when you will have to evacuate the salon quickly, for example if there was a fire. It is important that you know exactly what to do to make sure you are safe and also to make sure others in the salon are safe.

evacuate: leave to go to a safer place

There should be someone in the salon who will take charge in the event of an evacuation. This person may be called a fire marshal, but you must also know the procedure to follow. All fire exits should be clearly marked.

TRY IT OUT!

If you don't already know or are not sure, find out exactly where the fire exits are in the salon where you work so you could act quickly if it becomes necessary.

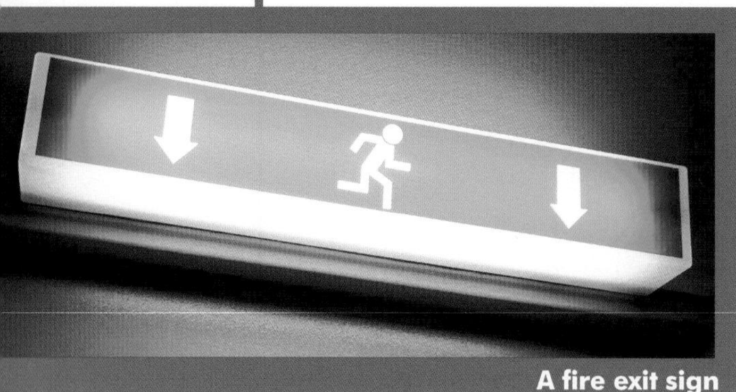
A fire exit sign

When evacuating the salon, leave quickly without running. Don't stop to take your personal belongings such as a coat or mobile phone, as this will put you at risk because it will take you longer to get out of the salon.

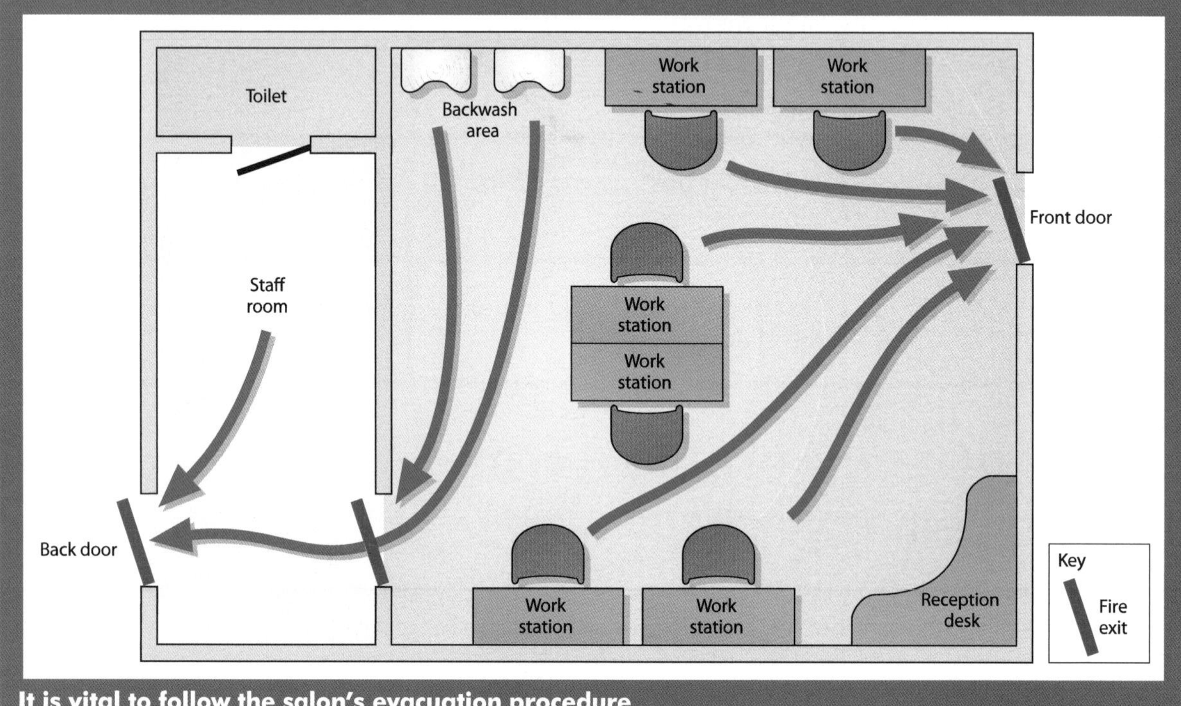

It is vital to follow the salon's evacuation procedure

You must know where to go when you have evacuated the salon. There will be an assembly point outside the building where everyone who has evacuated the salon will meet. This is to ensure that everyone can be accounted for. If anyone is missing, the fire service can then be told and fire fighters will enter the building to try to find the missing person. If you decided to go home, the fire marshal would not know where you were and fire fighters could risk their lives trying to find you.

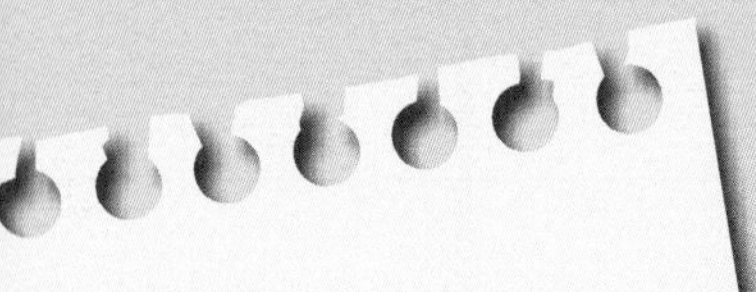

OVER TO YOU...

Draw a simple plan of the salon where you work and mark on it:

- The fire exits.
- The assembly point.

It is a good idea to know where the fire fighting equipment is kept if a minor fire breaks out. There are different types of fire extinguisher to be used on different types of fire. It is important that you know what type of fire each extinguisher should be used on – see the table below. All fire extinguishers should now be mainly red coloured, with a zone or area of colour that tells you what the different content of the extinguisher is.

small

Types of fire extinguisher

Extinguisher	Uses	Do not use on
Water	For wood, paper, textile and solid material fires	Liquid, electrical or metal fires
Powder	For liquid and electrical fires	Metal fires
Foam	For liquid fires	Electrical or metal fires
Carbon dioxide	For liquid and electrical fires	Metal fires

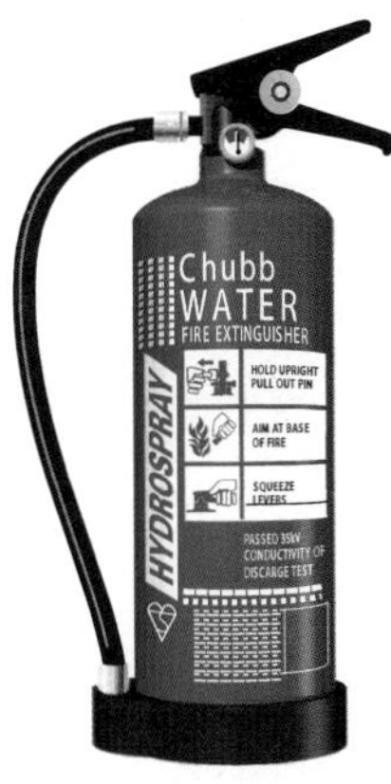

Water

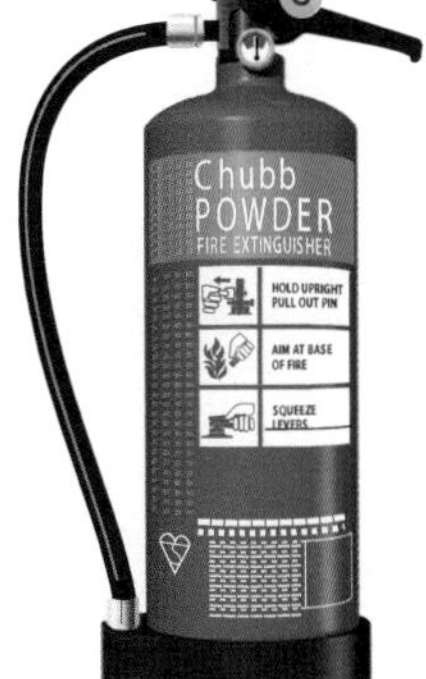

Powder

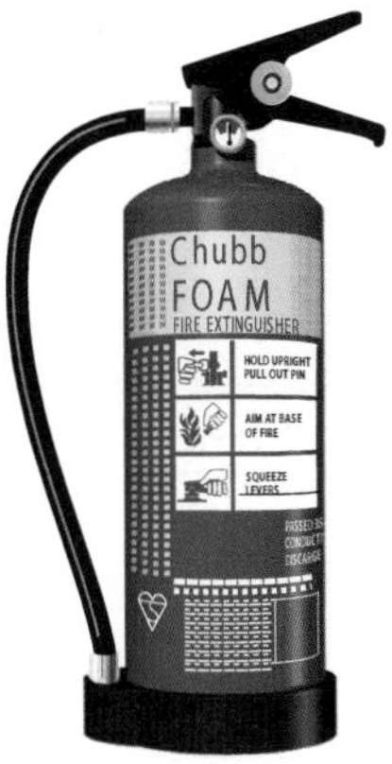

Foam

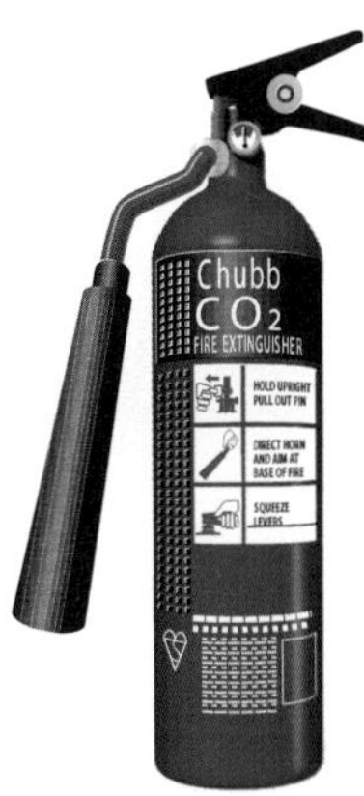

Carbon dioxide

Fire extinguishers

If you use the wrong type of extinguisher on a fire, you could make the fire much worse and/or cause serious injuries to yourself or someone else. For example, if you try to put out an electrical fire with a water extinguisher, you could be electrocuted.

OVER TO YOU...

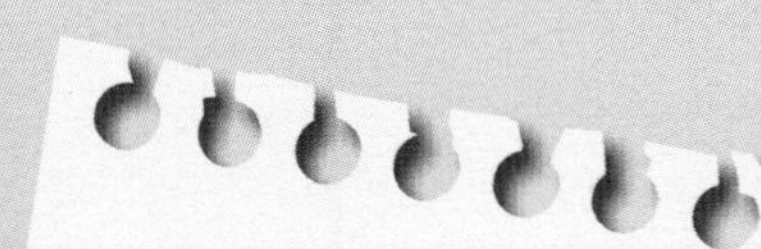

Which fire extinguishers can be used on:

- Electrical fires?
- Non-electrical fires?

Fire blankets can also be used to smother flames. They are especially good for wrapping around someone who is on fire. Fire blankets may also be used after using either a powder or carbon dioxide extinguisher. Both of these extinguishers will put out a fire, but they don't cool it down, so the fire could start up again. The fire blanket makes sure this doesn't happen again.

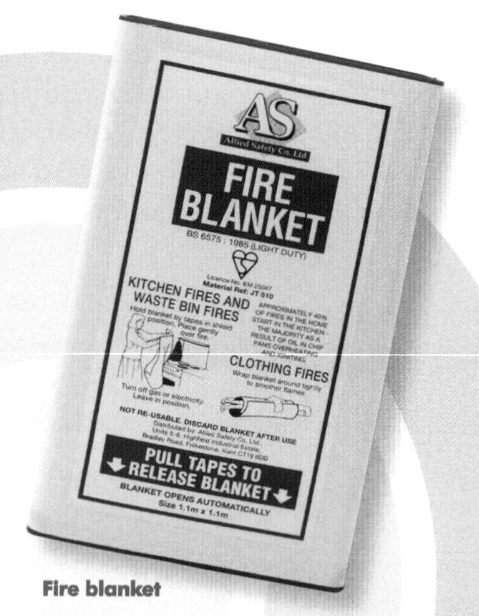

Fire blanket

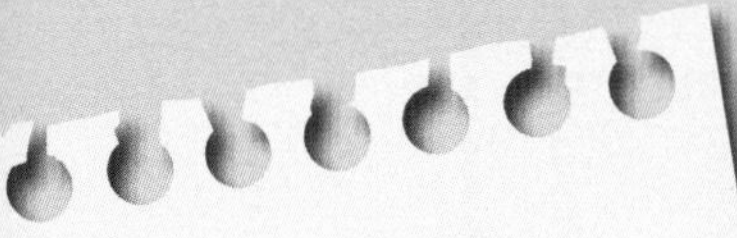

OVER TO YOU...

On the plan of the salon's fire exits and assembly point that you made earlier, mark the location of:

- Fire extinguishers, using the colour codes of each extinguisher.
- The fire blanket.
- The first aid kit.

This will help you to remember where equipment is kept.

Check what you know...

1. A hazard is:

- [ ] a piece of paper that tells you the rules of the salon
- [ ] something you can do to stop people in the salon from getting hurt
- [ ] something that could possibly cause an accident or an injury

2. You shouldn't use a hairdryer or wax pot if:

- [ ] it is nice and clean
- [ ] it is switched on
- [ ] the flex (wire) is frayed

3. Which of the following can be used to sterilise your tools?

- [ ] sting rays
- [ ] supersonic rays
- [ ] ultra-violet rays

4. The temperature in the salon should be:

- [ ] 14 – 16°C
- [ ] 18 – 21°C
- [ ] 25 – 31°C

5. Aerosols shouldn't be stored on a sunny window ledge because:

- [ ] they might change colour
- [ ] the product inside the aerosol won't work properly afterwards
- [ ] it might explode

6. When should you report minor accidents at work?

- [ ] when you have a minute
- [ ] as soon as you possibly can
- [ ] you don't need to report minor accidents

7. Hydraulic couches and beds are useful because:

- [ ] they make the salon look very professional
- [ ] they help to stop you bending and getting backache
- [ ] they come in a variety of different colours

8. If you notice some boxes blocking the fire exit, what should you do?

- [ ] move them immediately
- [ ] tell one of the clients about the boxes
- [ ] nothing, they'll be OK there

9. A fire blanket can be used to:

- [ ] keep you warm
- [ ] keep a fire going
- [ ] smother a fire

10. When evacuating the salon in the event of a fire, should you stop to get your mobile phone?

- [ ] yes, you might need to phone your mum or dad
- [ ] no, you might end up being trapped in the fire
- [ ] yes, it cost a lot of money and it shouldn't be left to burn in the fire

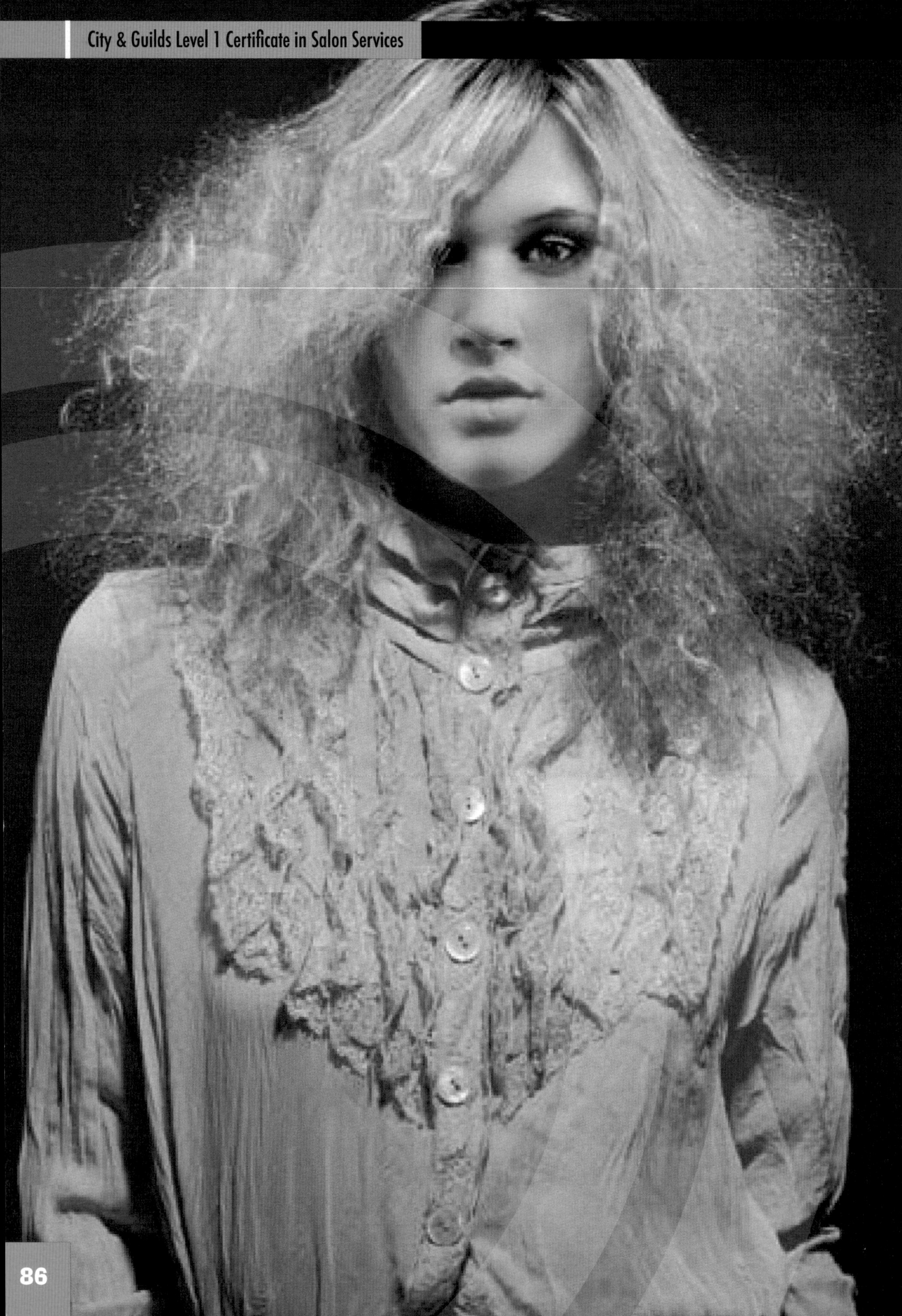

Unit 5

Hairdressing services

This is an exciting unit as it introduces a variety of hairdressing skills. There are lots of practical hairdressing activities for you to do and also some very important knowledge you must learn. The practical activities and the theory together will make sure you can work safely and successfully.

In this unit you will learn about:

- The basic structure of the hair.
- Preparing the client for hairdressing services.
- Hair, skin and scalp conditions.
- Shampooing and conditioning the hair and scalp.
- Blow-drying, setting and styling.
- Plaiting and braiding.

Towards the end of this course, you will be observed and assessed on:

- Preparing for basic services.
- Shampooing and conditioning the hair and scalp.
- Drying and finishing hair using basic techniques.

The basic structure of the hair

You need to know a bit about hair before you can work with it. You need to understand what it does and how this may affect the hairdressing services you are going to carry out.

make you change

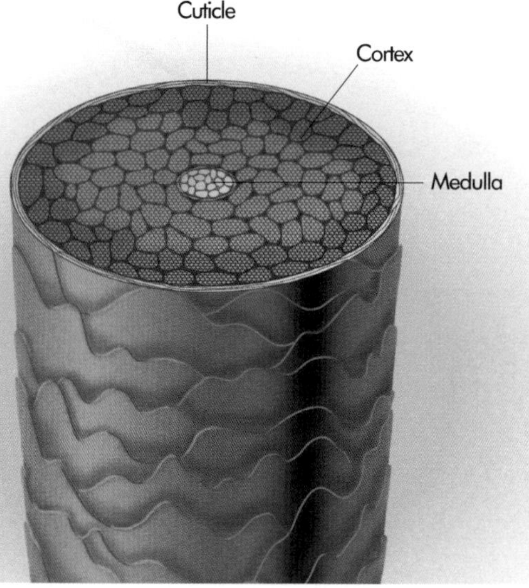

The three layers of the hair

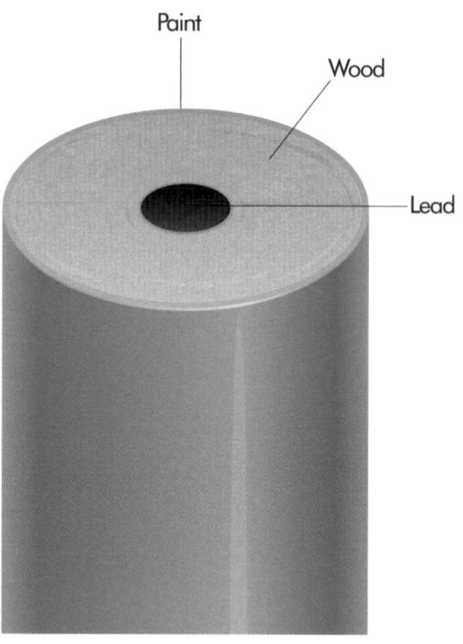

The three layers of the hair are a bit like the three parts of a pencil

The hair has three layers:

1 The outside layer of the hair is called the **cuticle**. It is made up from layers of overlapping scale-like bands – although you can't see these, they look a bit like fish scales. The cuticle protects the inside parts of the hair, but it can become damaged by harsh treatment, e.g. overuse of colours or straightening irons (if they're used incorrectly).
2 The **cortex** is the next layer of the hair. It makes up the largest part of the hair. It consists of lots of bunches of parallel fibres, a bit like holding a handful of drinking straws. This part of the hair is important because it is where the colouring, perming and relaxing processes take place.
3 The **medulla** is in the centre of the hair. It is made up of small cells with air spaces in between. It does not affect any of the hairdressing services you will do; in fact, some people don't even have one!

side by side

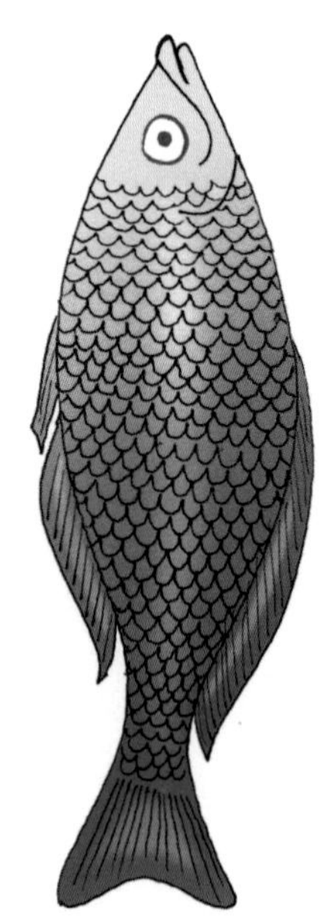

The cuticle layer looks a bit like fish scales

Preparing the client for hairdressing services

It is important to make sure the client is properly prepared and protected ready for the hairdressing service that is to take place.

Preparing a trolley for salon services

It is important that you prepare everything you might need for the salon service before the client arrives. Twenty minutes before, make sure all your tools are being sterilised. All work areas should be wiped down and mirrors and chairs cleaned. You can then set up your trolley for the service your client is having.

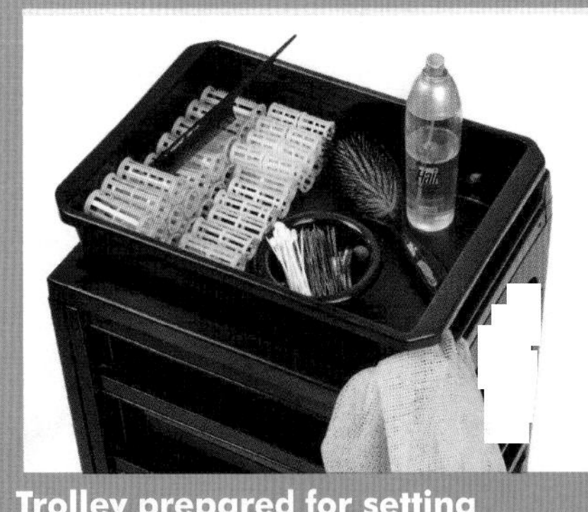

Trolley prepared for setting

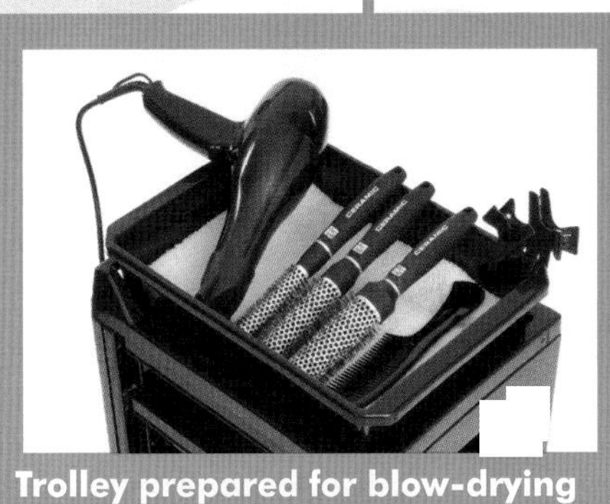

Trolley prepared for blow-drying

Once the trolley is ready, store any personal belongings such as your bag safely where they cannot be seen and no one will trip over them.

Equipment

The client must always wear a gown to protect his or her clothing from any spillages, for example water, colouring products, hair products and so on.

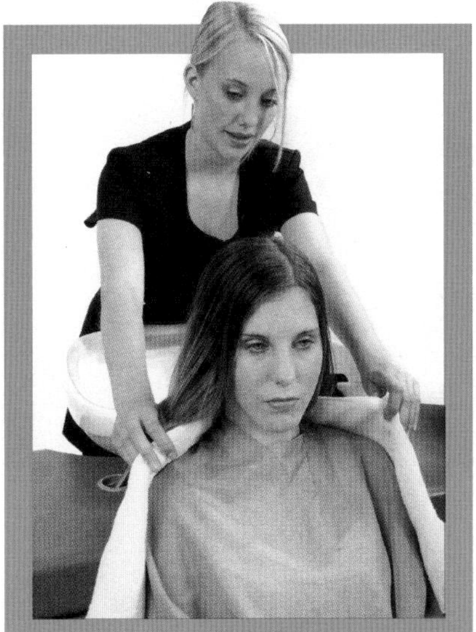

A client being prepared for a hairdressing service

A towel around the client's shoulders will also help to protect clothes from spillages. It should keep the client dry as it will absorb water and products dripping from the hair.

Cotton wool is used during the perming process to protect the hairline from the chemicals used when perming hair. It may also be used to protect the client's ears while they are under the hood dryer.

Tissues are used to help protect the client's gown and keep it clean – tuck a tissue around the back of the gown where the neck is.

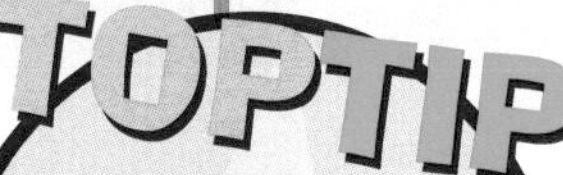

If the client's towel becomes wet, you should change it for a dry one immediately. This will help the client to stay comfortable throughout the service.

TOPTIP

Protect the client's ears under the hood dryer by rolling cotton wool into a spiral and tucking it underneath the hair net making sure the ears are covered.

How to prepare a client for a hairdressing service (gown and towel)

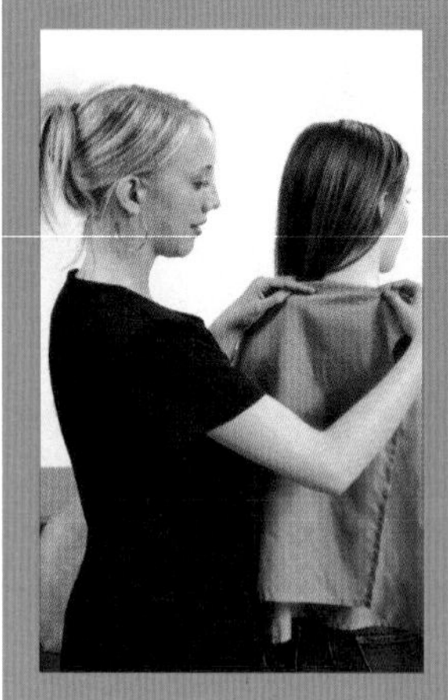

1 Gown the client to protect her clothing.

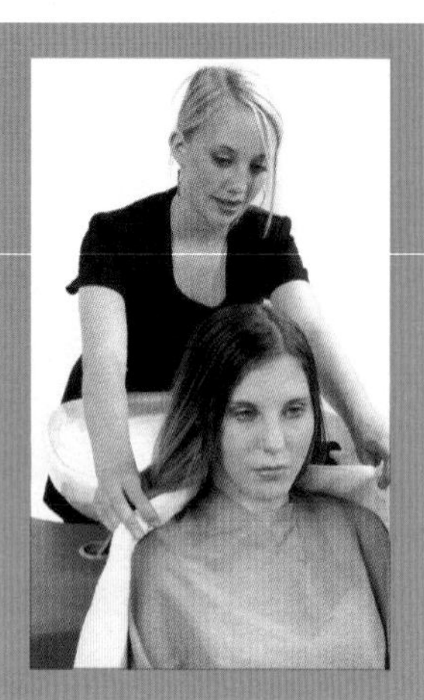

2 Place a towel around the client's shoulders.

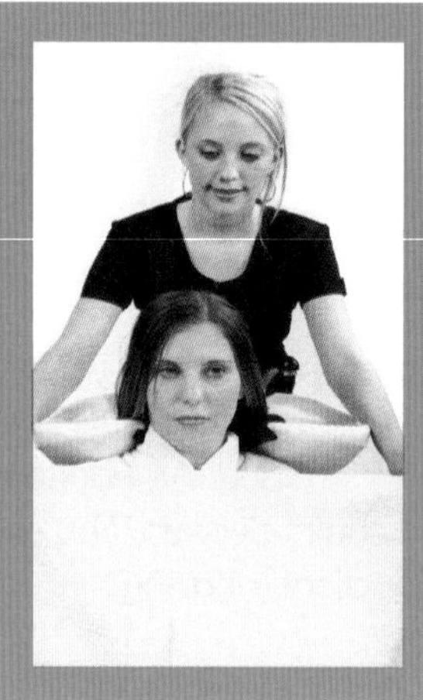

3 Place a towel around the front of the client.

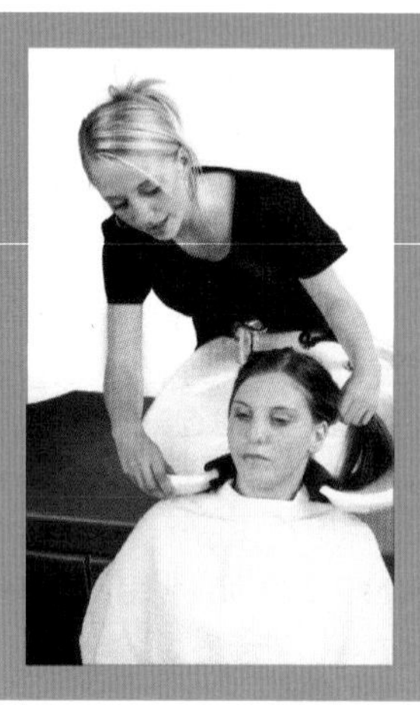

4 Position the client at the backwash making any adjustments that are necessary to ensure the client is comfortable.

salon scene

Tania was training to be a hairdresser. Every Wednesday evening was model night, when she was allowed to bring in her own models and either learn something new or practise something she had done before. The previous few days had been really hot and today it was not only very hot but also very humid. Tania's friend Casey was coming into the salon as Tania wanted to practise using curling tongs. When Casey arrived Tania went to gown her up, but Casey said it was far too hot to wear a gown. As Tania was not going to be using any products, nothing would spill onto her clothes, and so she decided Casey would not need a gown.

Tania was getting on well with her tonging technique despite the fact the salon was very warm and her hands were sweaty. Suddenly, the tongs slipped out of Tania's hands and landed on Casey's arm. Casey screamed out in pain and Tania quickly removed the tongs from her friend's arm, but too late ... the tongs had left a large burn.

What went wrong?

Would you have done things differently if you were Tania?

Hairdressing products for different conditions

You will need to be able to identify what hair condition each client has. With the help of your tutor, you should be able to tell the difference between dry, normal, greasy and dandruff affected hair:

- Dry hair often feels dry and sometimes a bit rough to the touch. It usually lacks shine.
- Greasy hair looks oily, especially at the roots of the hair. As it is oily, it can look shiny.
- Normal hair feels smooth to the touch and generally looks shiny and healthy.
- The scalp of dandruff affected hair is usually dry and flaky and is sometimes itchy.

scalp: the skin on the head under the hair

Most children have normal hair – when the hair is brushed it looks silky and smooth. When you become a teenager (or slightly before) your body changes and starts to produce more oil, which is why most teenagers have greasy hair and skin.

There are several reasons why hair may become dry. Here are the most common ones:

- Overuse of chemicals on the hair, e.g. colours or bleach.
- Incorrect use of heated styling appliances, e.g. straightening irons, will cause the hair to become dry and brittle.
- Being out in the strong sunlight or wind.

brittle: easily broken

It is important to find out all about the client's hair before you start shampooing. This information should be written onto a consultation sheet.

Shampoo Service Consultation Sheet

Student's name ______________________

Client's name ______________________

Date ______________________

Client's hair condition:
- ☐ Dry
- ☐ Normal
- ☐ Greasy
- ☐ Dandruff affected

Hair length:
- ☐ Long
- ☐ Medium
- ☐ Short

Has the client's hair been coloured, permed or relaxed?
- ☐ Coloured
- ☐ Permed
- ☐ Relaxed

Which shampoo should be used?
____

Which conditioner should be used?
____

Consultation sheet for a shampooing service

Hair, skin and scalp conditions

It is important that you analyse the client's hair, skin and scalp before carrying out any hairdressing service. This is because the client may have a condition that would stop the service from going ahead or maybe the service could still be done but with extreme care. You will need to know which hair, skin and scalp conditions will contra-indicate the service.

examine

medical problem

a reason why something shouldn't be done

Hair conditions

While you are chatting to the client, you should be looking at the client's hair and scalp. You will need to do this discreetly so the client thinks you are just feeling the hair. You should be checking for head lice or nits (eggs). These are usually found in the nape of the neck and behind the ears, but you should check all over as they could be anywhere on the scalp.

secretly

If you find the client has head lice or nits, you should inform your tutor immediately (but discreetly) as the client will not be able to have the service until the head lice have been treated.

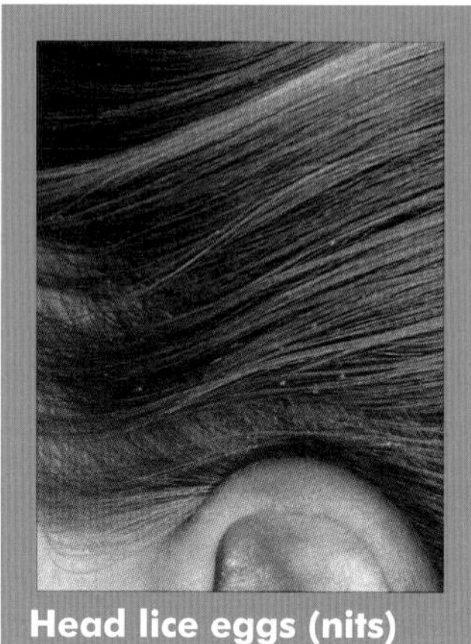

Head lice eggs (nits)

Skin conditions and scalp conditions

If a client has open cuts and abrasions on the scalp, hair products may get into the cuts and cause discomfort to the client. There is also the risk of the open cuts becoming infected.

scrapes

As well as looking for head lice, you must make sure the skin and scalp are suitable for the hairdressing service.

Sometimes clients may have areas on their skin or scalp that are red and swollen. This would usually be because they have an infection (or the beginning of one) or because they have a skin disorder such as eczema, in which case it may be sore.

You need to look closely to see if the area has evidence of pus (you can tell this because it will be yellow, like really bad spots), which could mean the client has a bacterial infection which may then be passed to other people. An example of this would be the skin condition, impetigo.

If you do not realise (or properly check) that the client has a skin or scalp condition, or an infestation, this could lead to cross infection.

large numbers of insects or organisms

Sterilisation

To prevent the risk of cross infection, tools and equipment used in the salon should be clean and sterile. It is good practice to sterilise your tools after each client.

free from germs

To remind yourself of the different methods of sterilisation, look back at Unit 4 Health and safety, page 69.

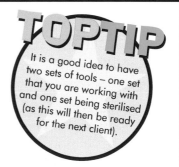

TOPTIP
It is a good idea to have two sets of tools – one set that you are working with and one set being sterilised (as this will then be ready for the next client).

Shampooing and conditioning the hair and scalp

Products, equipment and materials

It is important that you know the right products to use when shampooing and conditioning hair as this will help you to get the best result possible. Shampoo is designed to clean the hair and scalp, while the conditioner's job is to smooth down the cuticles and make the hair easier to comb. The table below shows the products, tools and equipment you will need to carry out this service.

Products, tools and equipment used when shampooing and conditioning hair

Products, tools and equipment	Why they are used
Shampoo	To thoroughly clean the hair and scalp – to remove dirt, grease and products. To prepare the hair for other services, e.g. blow-drying or setting.
Conditioner	To smooth the cuticles and help to disentangle the hair. To add shine to the hair.
Frontwash	Used to shampoo the hair.
Backwash	Used to shampoo the hair. Especially good for long hair.
Rake comb	Used to disentangle the hair.

untangle

Shampoos and conditioners

As each client's hair is different, it is important to use the correct hair products for different hair conditions – see the table below.

Products for use on different hair conditions

Hair condition	Correct shampoo to use	Correct conditioner to use
Dry	Cream or oil-based, e.g. coconut shampoo	Surface conditioner or leave-in conditioner
Normal	Fruit-based, rosemary or any thing suitable for normal hair	Surface conditioner or leave-in conditioner
Greasy	Citrus-based shampoo, e.g. lemon, lime	Surface conditioner (only on the ends of the hair if it's dry; keep the conditioner away from the root area as it may make the hair more greasy)
Dandruff affected	Medicated shampoo	Surface conditioner or hot oil treatment

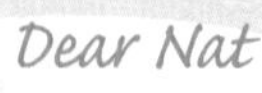

Dear Nat

My boss keeps going on about using the right kind of shampoo for the client's hair. Is there really a right kind of shampoo, or are they all the same but with different colours and smells?

From Rachel

Nat says

Your boss is right! There really is a right shampoo for each client's hair. Shampoos for different hair conditions have different ingredients because they have different jobs to do. For example, a shampoo for dry and damaged hair will contain ingredients to add moisture to the hair and help to make it strong and healthy again. If you used shampoo like this on greasy hair, it would make the hair even greasier!

TRY IT OUT!

Find out the names of all the shampoos and conditioners in the salon where you work. Then make a chart so you can see which shampoos and conditioners are best for different hair conditions.

Massage movements

Before you begin to shampoo hair, you need to know the massage movements needed so that you will be able to give a good shampooing service. Shampooing is very important as it prepares the hair for the following service. If it is done well, it can make the client feel relaxed, ready to enjoy the rest of the service.

TOP TIP
A badly done shampoo will leave you with an unhappy client and possibly an unhappy stylist too!

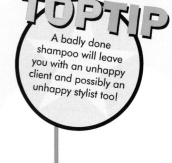

Effleurage – this is the massage movement you should use to apply both shampoo and conditioner. It is a smooth stroking movement that starts at the front of the head and covers the entire scalp.

Rotary – this is the rubbing movement you do when you shampoo the hair. Rotary should be carried out in a methodical way, using the pads of your fingers and working in small round movements over the scalp.

methodical: following a pattern

Petrissage – this is the massage movement you should use when you condition the hair. It is quite like rotary (as you still do a methodical massage in small round movements, using the pads of your fingers), but it is a much slower and firmer movement. You will know if you are pressing hard enough because you should see the client's forehead move up and down.

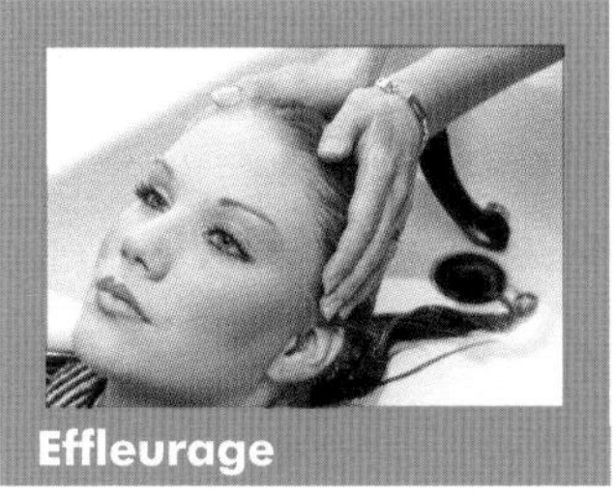
Effleurage

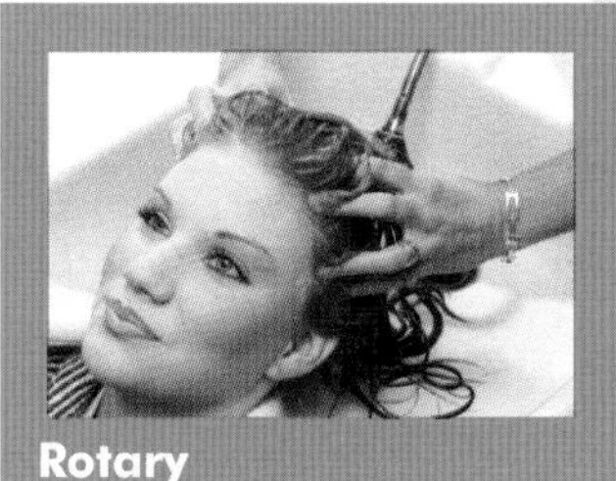
Rotary

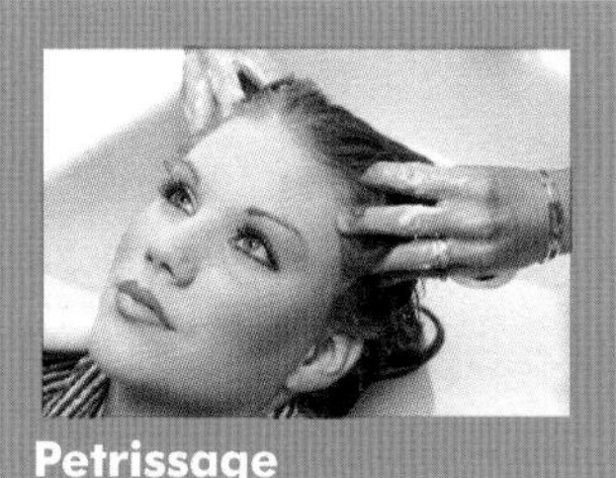
Petrissage

Positioning the client for shampooing

Frontwash or backwash?

Some clients will have a preference, but for others, before deciding on a front or backwash, you should think about the following:

- Is the client wearing make-up? If so, a backwash would be better.
- Does the client mind if her make-up is washed off? If not, then you can use either.
- If the client wants a frontwash, give them a towel to protect their face.
- Is the client's hair very long? If so, a backwash would be better as the hair will not get in the way of the client's face while you are shampooing.
- Does the client have back or neck problems? If so, then a frontwash might be better. It is a good idea to check this with the client during your consultation.

You will need to make sure the client is comfortable throughout the shampooing and conditioning service. Your client's comfort will depend on his or her position at the basin. You may need to adjust the position of the chair to make sure the basin is at the right height. Some salons have specially designed, soft neck rests (sometimes called 'rubber necks') on the backwash to make the client more comfortable. Before you start to shampoo, check with the client that he or she is comfortable.

There may be serious problems if the client is wrongly positioned, especially at the backwash. If there is too much pressure put onto the back of the neck, this could lead to the client having a stroke! Less serious problems could be the client getting wet and then being uncomfortable.

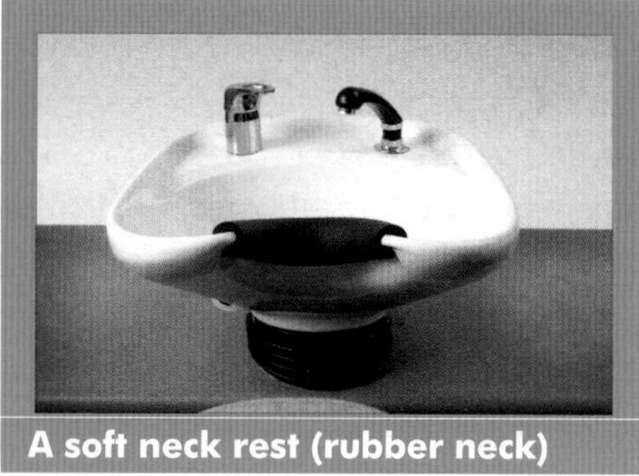

A soft neck rest (rubber neck)

Dear Nat

I've just started work in a hairdressing salon and I'm really enjoying it. I love shampooing the clients' hair and having a chat. The only problem is some of the clients complain that their neck hurts when they've had their hair shampooed at the backwash. Am I doing something wrong or do some clients just like moaning?

From Sophia

Nat says

Yes, some clients do like to moan, but I think the problem may be because you haven't positioned them properly at the backwash. Perhaps you could offer them a frontwash (if they are available in your salon). Ask your boss or tutor to show you how they should be positioned to make sure they are comfortable. It may be useful to use a specially designed, soft neck rest on the basin.

Shampooing hair

When shampooing the client's hair, make sure you have the water flow and temperature right. If there is not enough water coming out of the shower head, it will take you a long time to rinse the shampoo and conditioner out of the hair. If the flow is too fast, the water may spray everywhere and wet the client. The water needs to flow fast enough to rinse the hair thoroughly but not so fast as to wet the salon!

If the water is too cold, it may shock the client and it will not clean the hair properly, but if the water is too hot, it may burn the client's scalp.

You must also check the temperature of the water before you put it near the client's head. Do this by testing the water on the back of your hand or the inside of your wrist. If the water temperature feels all right on your hand, then it should be fine. Remember to check with the client that the temperature is comfortable for them.

TOPTIP

Remember to turn the water off while you are shampooing, as this will save water and money.

The client's hair should be thoroughly wet before you apply the shampoo. When you are using professional shampoos, you may be surprised at how little you will need to use. You should aim for one squirt from the shampoo dispenser. The hair may not lather up very well on the first shampoo, but don't worry, it will on the second (unless the hair is really dirty).

How to shampoo the hair

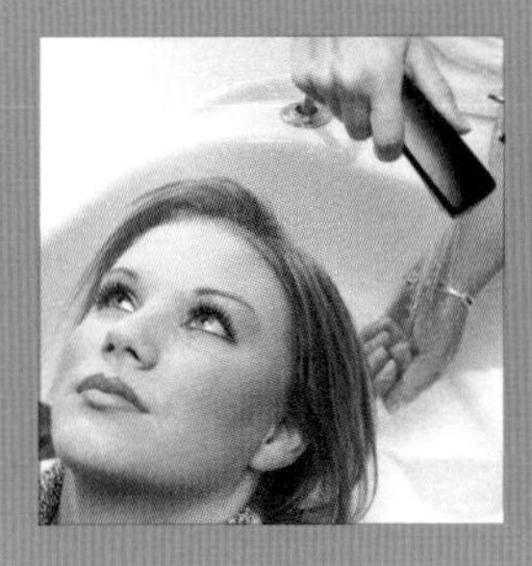

1 Test the water temperature on the inside of your wrist.

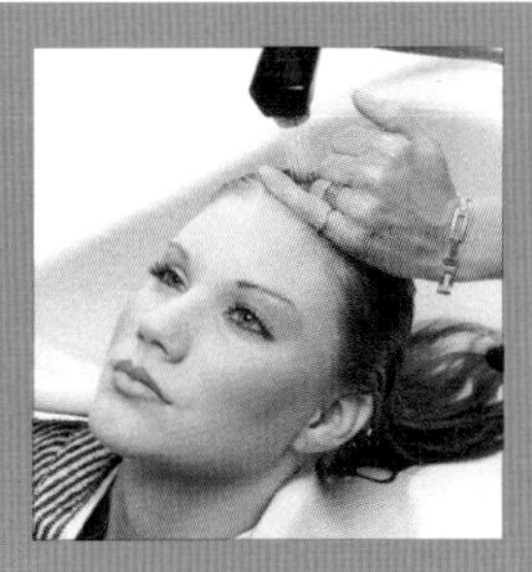

2 Check the temperature with the client. Thoroughly wet the hair and scalp. Turn off the water.

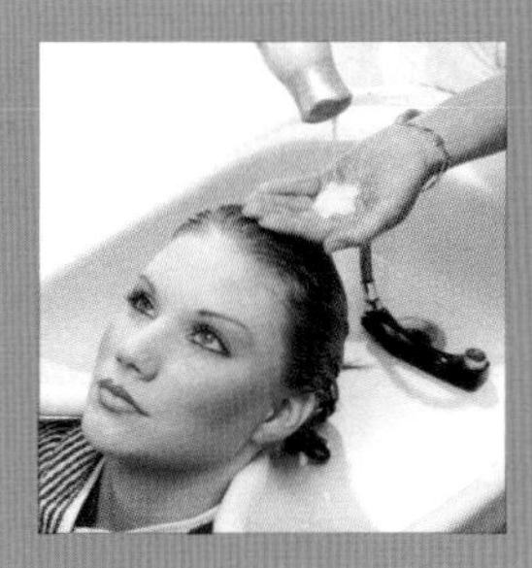

3 Squeeze a small amount of shampoo into the palm of your hand and smooth between both palms. Apply the shampoo using effleurage.

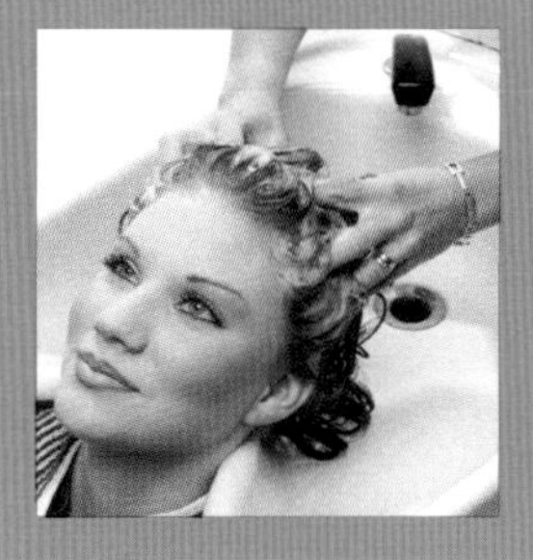

4 Use rotary massage until the whole head has been covered and the shampoo begins to lather.

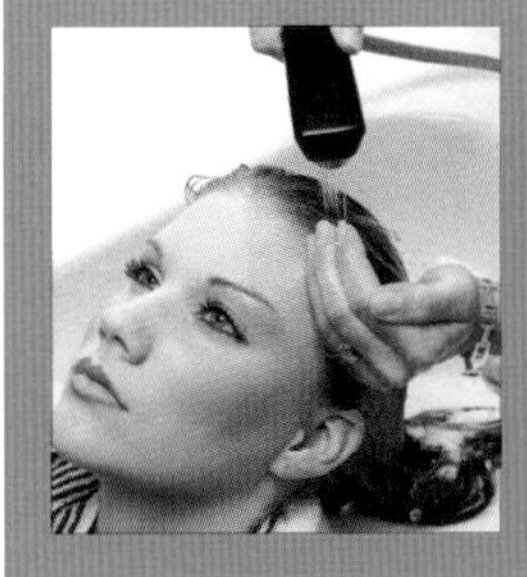

5 Rinse off the shampoo thoroughly. Now give the client's hair a second shampoo, repeating the process as for the first shampoo. When you have rinsed off the second shampoo, gently squeeze the hair to remove excess water.

salon scene

It was Taha's first day working in the hairdressing salon. He had been shown how to shampoo hair and had watched and listened closely during the demonstration. He really wanted to get it right.

When the next client came in, it was his turn to shampoo. Taha gowned the client and took her over to the backwash. He sat the client down, placed the towels as he had been shown and then asked the client to lean back into the backwash. The client placed her head into the basin and Taha began to wet the client's hair. The client sat up quickly complaining that it was too cold. As she sat up, the water shot straight down her back. In his panic Taha did not turn off the water and it kept running down the client's back, soaking her towel and gown.

One of the other staff members came to the rescue and finished shampooing the client's hair, but by this time the client's clothes were soaking wet!

What were all the things that Taha did wrong?

Conditioners

Conditioners are used to improve the condition of the hair by closing and smoothing the cuticles, adding shine to the hair and replacing moisture.

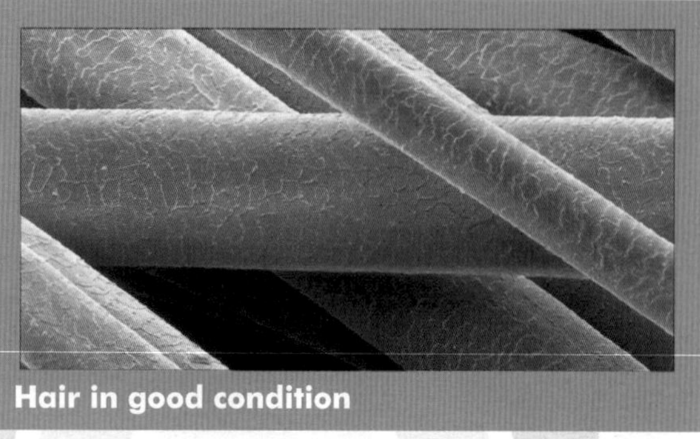
Hair in good condition

How to condition the hair

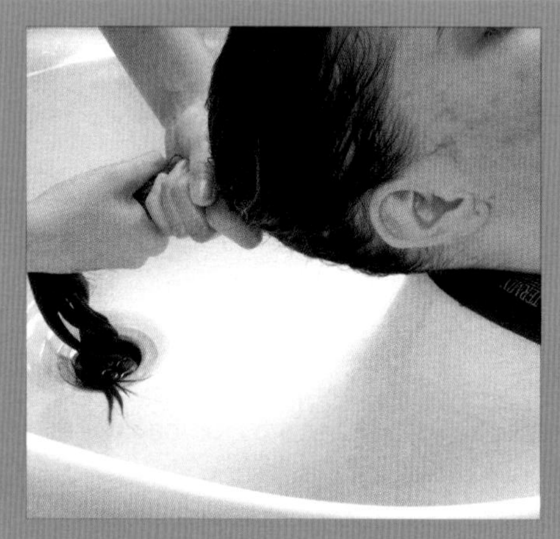

1 After rinsing the shampoo out of the hair, squeeze out all the excess water. (The water should be turned off.)

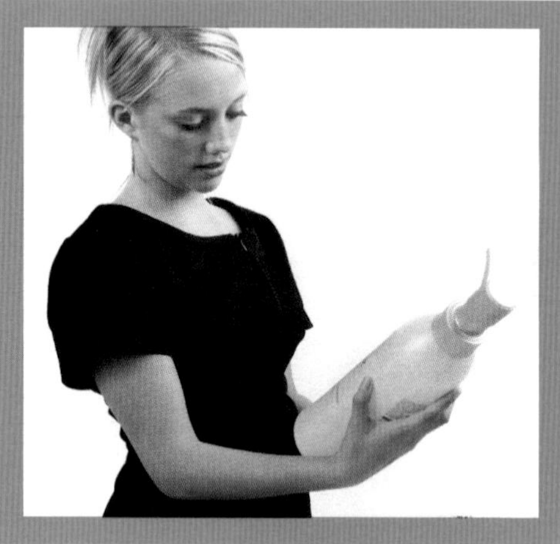

2 Choose the right conditioner for the client.

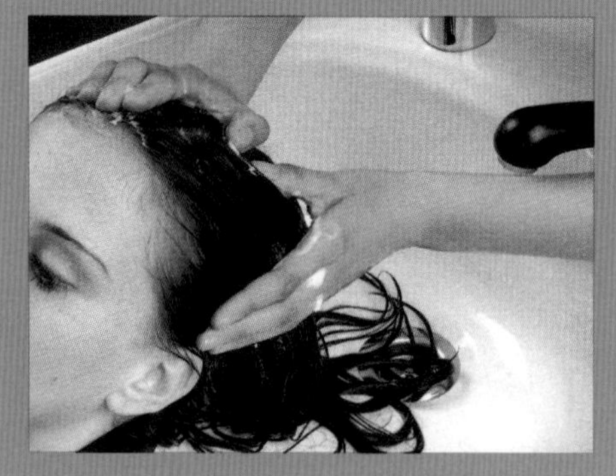

3 Apply the conditioner using the effleurage massage movement and then massage the scalp using petrissage. Do this for a couple of minutes or following the manufacturer's instructions.

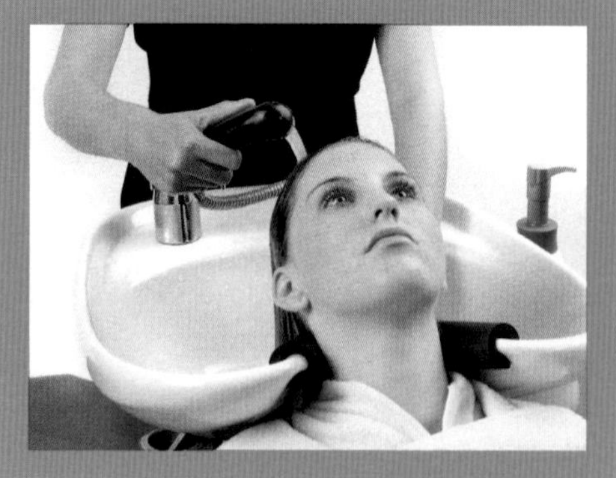

4 Turn on the water. Rinse the hair thoroughly to make sure you remove all the conditioner. If you don't, the hair will look lank and greasy and it will be hard to style. Turn off the water.

How to wrap and dry the hair

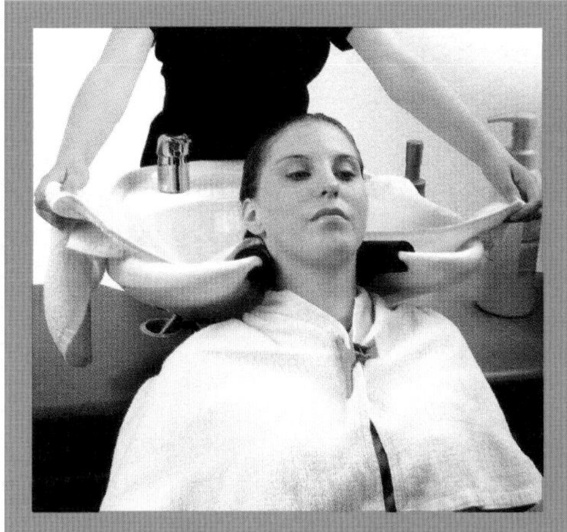

1 Take a towel and place at the back of the head.

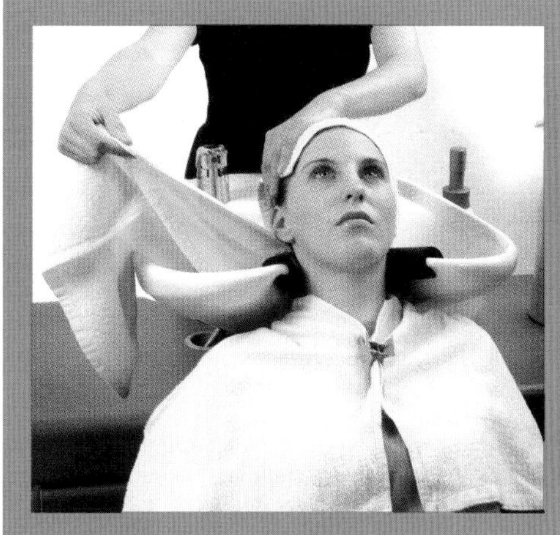

2 Take one side of the towel across, then the other.

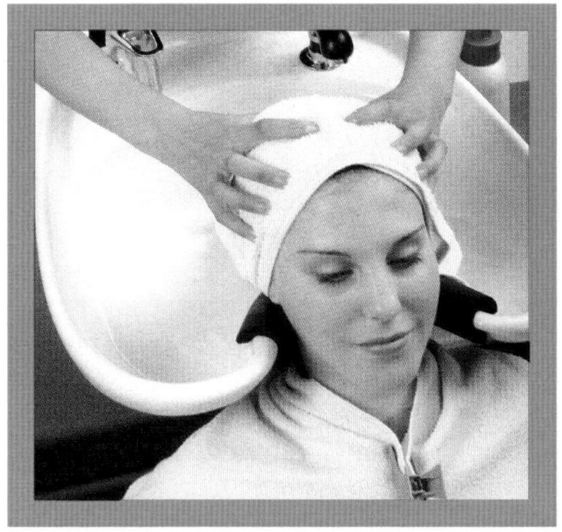

3 Gently press the towel against the hair to remove excess moisture.

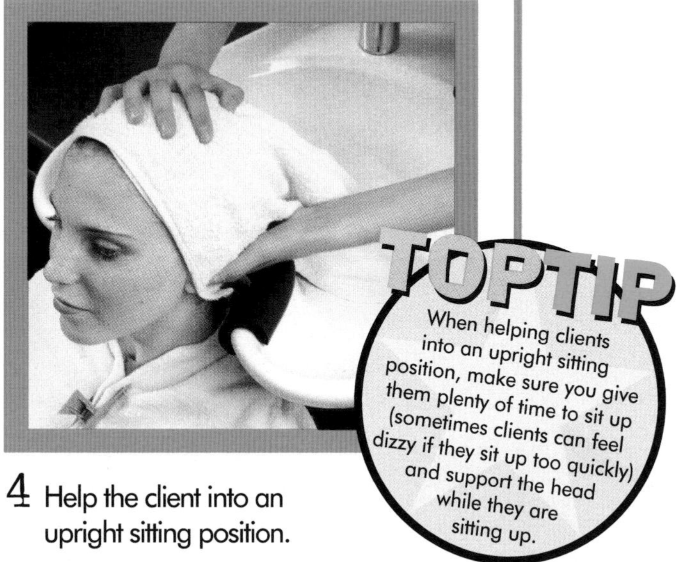

4 Help the client into an upright sitting position.

TOPTIP

When helping clients into an upright sitting position, make sure you give them plenty of time to sit up (sometimes clients can feel dizzy if they sit up too quickly) and support the head while they are sitting up.

Clean and tidy the work area

At the end of the service, you must make sure the basin area is left clean and tidy ready for the next person. The next client will not want to come to a dirty basin full of someone else's hair and shampoo everywhere! Cleaning and tidying also helps to stop cross infection.

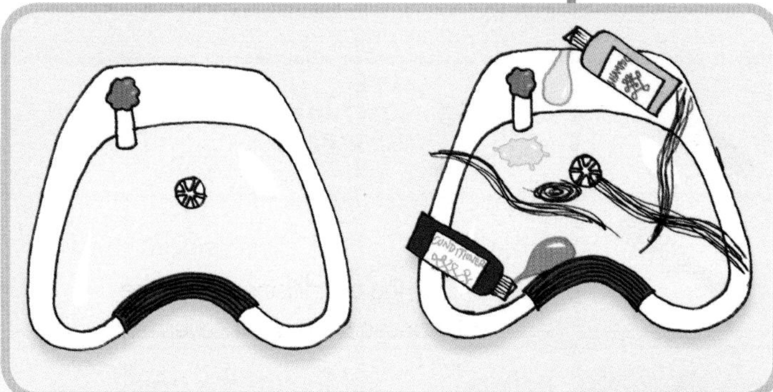

Which basin would you prefer to use?

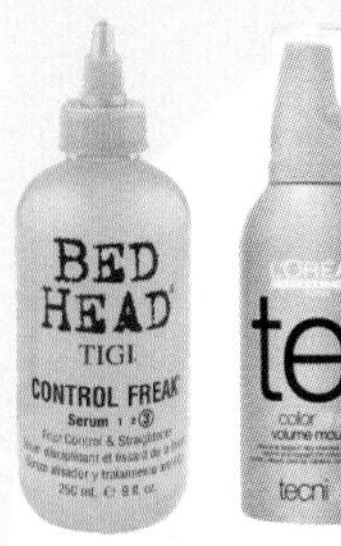

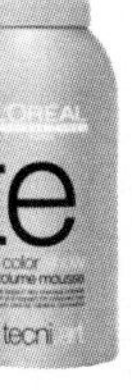

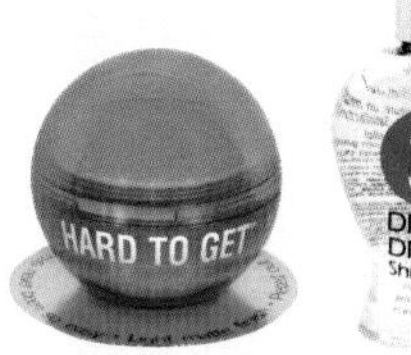

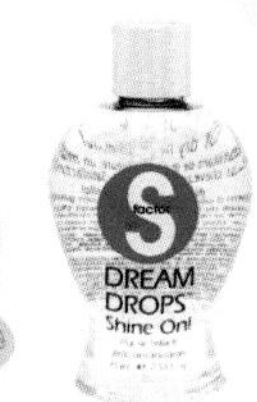

Styling products

Blow-drying, setting and styling

Styling products

Blow-dries and sets will stay in longer if you use styling products. They come in different strengths, depending how much hold the hair needs. For example, if the hair needs maximum hold, gel would be good to use as it is usually a very firm styling product.

TRY IT OUT!

With the help of your tutor, find out what styling products are available in the salon.

When you feel confident about blow-drying, section your block into four, as shown, and apply a different product to each section and blow-dry the hair.

Write down your results and keep them for future reference. Some of them were probably easier to use than others!

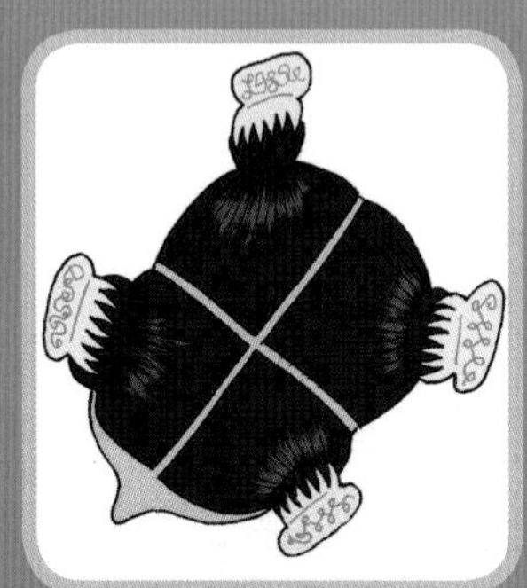

Hair sectioned into four

Basic hairdressing equipment

all pics to be cut-out if layout approved	Piece of equipment	Why is it used?	When is it used?	How is it sterilised/ cleaned?
	Tail comb	To take really straight sections	Setting	Chemical jar or UV cabinet
	Pin tail comb	To take really straight sections	Perming or braiding	Chemical jar or UV cabinet
	Dressing comb	To smooth and blend the hair	Dressing out a set	Chemical jar or UV cabinet
	Rake comb	To disentangle the hair	After shampooing and conditioning	Chemical jar or UV cabinet
	Rollers	To curl the hair	During setting	Hot soapy water

	Piece of equipment	Why is it used?	When is it used?	How is it sterilised/ cleaned?
	Pins	To hold the rollers in place	During setting	
	Grips	To hold the hair in place	When putting hair up	
	Professional bands	To secure plaits/braids	During plaiting/ braiding	
	Butterfly clip	To hold hair you are not working with out of the way	When disentangling hair and blow-drying	Chemical jar or UV cabinet
	Round brush	To curl hair or straighten hair	Blow-drying	UV cabinet
	Paddle brush	To blow-dry hair smooth and straight	Blow-drying	UV cabinet
	Vent brush	To give the hair a more natural look	Blow-drying	UV cabinet
	Dressing out brush	To make sure you remove all the roller lines	Dressing out a set	UV cabinet
	Hand dryer	To dry the hair	For blow-drying hair	Unplug the dryer, then wipe over with an alcohol-based wipe
	Nozzle attachment	To direct the airflow from the dryer making it easier to blow-dry	When blow-drying	Unplug the dryer, then wipe over with an alcohol-based wipe

	Piece of equipment	Why is it used?	When is it used?	How is it sterilised/ cleaned?
	Diffuser attachment	For a naturally curly result	When blow-drying	Unplug the dryer, then wipe over with an alcohol-based wipe
	Hood dryer	To dry hair	To dry hair that has been set	Unplug the dryer, then wipe over with an alcohol-based wipe
	Neck brush	To remove any hair clippings	After cutting	UV cabinet
	Back mirror	To show clients the back of their hair	When the service is finished	Wipe with a damp cloth or use a mirror/window cleaning spray

Blow-drying the hair

Before blow-drying, make sure the hair has been thoroughly shampooed (and conditioned if needed). After you have towel dried, disentangle the hair carefully starting at the nape, at the points of the hair and work up to the roots.

towel dried: pressed on the towel while it is wrapped around the client's head

nape: the back/bottom of the hair, where it meets the neck

points: ends

If the hair is still very wet, you should blast it dry with the hairdryer. You can use the dryer without a nozzle to do this (as you don't need to control the hair in the same way as you do when blow-drying).

Sectioning the hair

It is important to divide the hair into neat, straight sections. This will make it much easier to blow-dry, as you will be able to see where you are working and will get a better result.

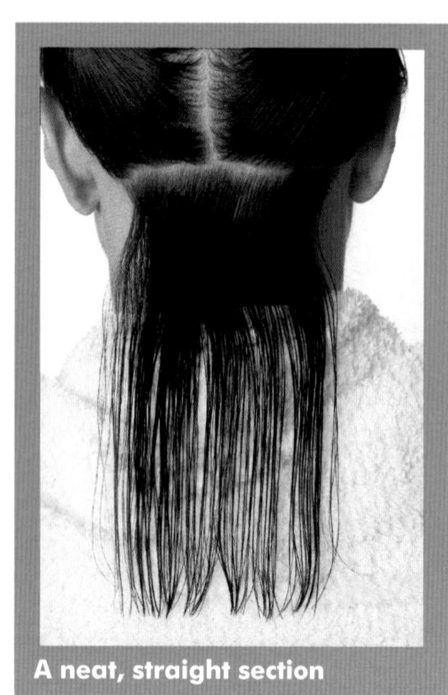

A neat, straight section

You must make sure you always direct the air flow from the blow-dryer down the hair (from roots to points), as this is the way the cuticle lies. Doing this will help the cuticles to lie flat and the hair will look shiny and healthy. You must also think about the temperature and speed setting on the blow-dryer.

Dry the roots of the hair first, being careful to keep your dryer moving so you don't burn the client's scalp (especially in the nape and around the ears). Then move on to the mid-lengths and ends. Check each section of the hair is thoroughly dry before you move onto the next section. As you bring each section down, be careful not to wet the sections you have already dried, so let the section drop and comb it smooth, away from the hair you have just dried.

TOP TIP

While you are learning, it is better to blow-dry the hair on the medium heat setting, as this will prevent you from over drying the hair and damaging the cuticles. You can tell hair that has been over dried as it looks dry and brittle and tends to be flyaway and hard to manage. By using the medium speed setting you will have more control over the hair while you are blow-drying.

Always blow-dry hair in the direction it will fall when the style is finished as this will:

- Make it easier to dress at the end.
- Make it last longer for the client.
- Make it easier for the client to manage.

TRY IT OUT!

Ask your tutor to show you how to blow-dry hair:

- Smooth and straight.
- Curly and bouncy.

Dear Nat

I have just started a hairdressing course and I'm learning to blow-dry. It doesn't matter how hard I pull the hair, I just can't get a really smooth finish. I don't want to hurt my clients, but I'm just not sure what to do.

From Nick

Nat says

You are quite right not to want to hurt your clients! You should always blow-dry with enough tension to get a smooth finish, but if you use too much tension, the hair may over stretch (especially if the hair isn't in very good condition). If the hair is over stretched, it will look uneven around the edges when you have finished. You should also make sure you use a nozzle on the hairdryer as this will direct the airflow and help to create a smooth finish.

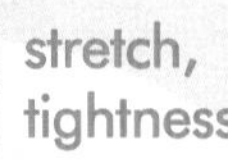
stretch, tightness

Ask your tutor to stay with you while you are blow-drying. Blow-dry a few sections first, then get your tutor to blow-dry a couple of sections. You can then ask the client how it felt, for example were you pulling as much as the tutor?

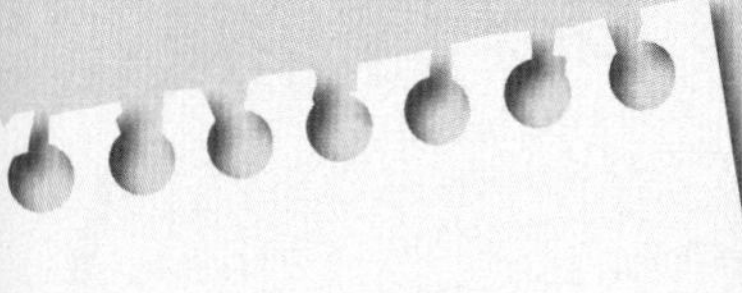

OVER TO YOU...

Find pictures of hair styles that can be achieved with blow-drying, with and without attachments. They could be from magazines or journals, photographs or sketches. Add them to your portfolio or scrapbook.

Finger drying the hair

This is best done on medium or short hair that has some natural movement. You must follow the same principles as you do for blow drying. The hair should be sectioned into neat, straight sections and the roots dried first. The big difference is that instead of using a brush to blow-dry the hair, you use your fingers.

natural movement: waves or curls; hair that is not straight

principles: rules

How to finger dry the hair

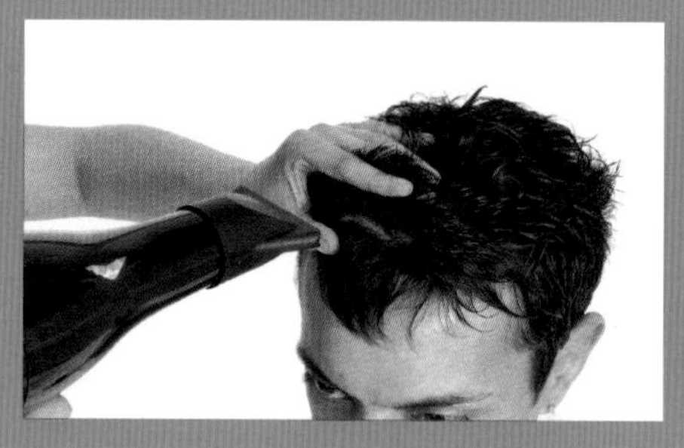

1 Lift the hair at the roots with your fingers (making sure the air flow is going from roots to points).

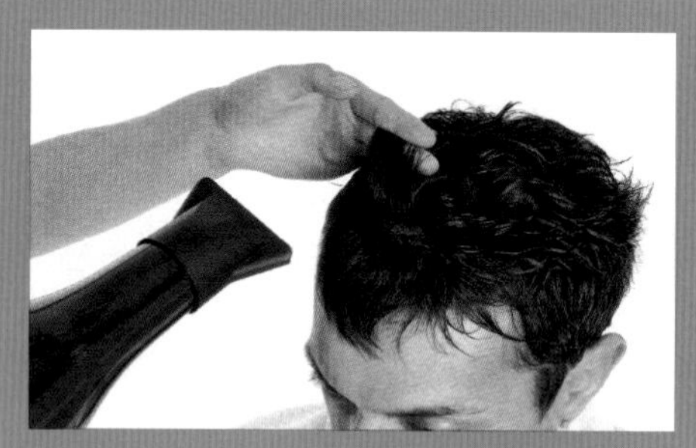

2 When the roots are dry, lift the rest of the hair and mould it into the direction you want the hair to fall.

When you have dried all the hair, either run your fingers through it to give it a textured look or use a vent brush, then add some wax to finish off.

textured: natural or non-styled

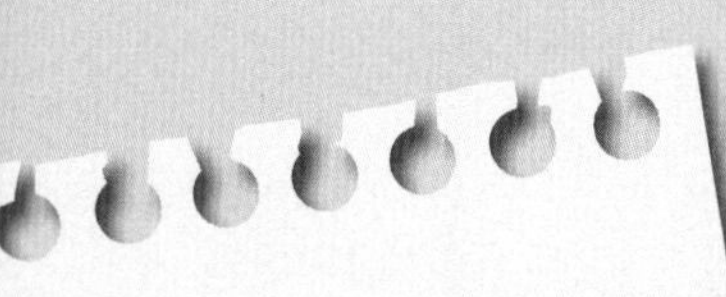

OVER TO YOU...

Find pictures of hair styles that can be achieved with finger drying. They could be from magazines or journals, photographs or sketches. Add them to your portfolio or scrapbook.

Setting the hair

Setting the hair will give root lift, curl and volume.

root lift: where the hair is bouncy at the roots

volume: where the hair looks fuller, 'big' hair

You can set hair using either ordinary rollers with pins, Velcro rollers that just stick in the hair or heated electric rollers with pins. Each of the different types of rollers comes in different sizes. The length of the client's hair and how curly the client wants it, will help you to decide what size roller to use. Big rollers will give a soft curl and are better to use on long hair, whereas small rollers will give a smaller, tighter curl on short hair.

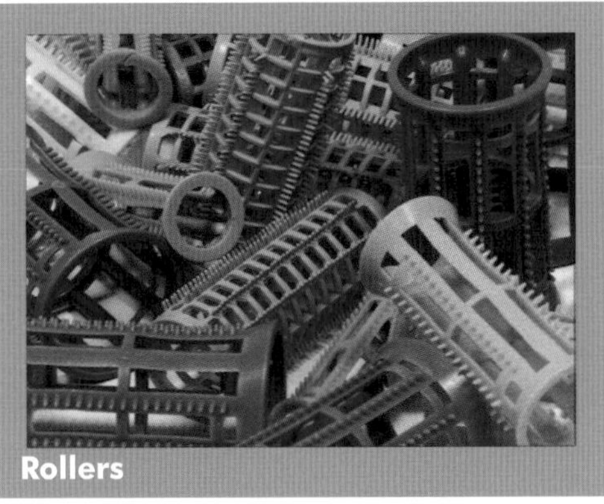
Rollers

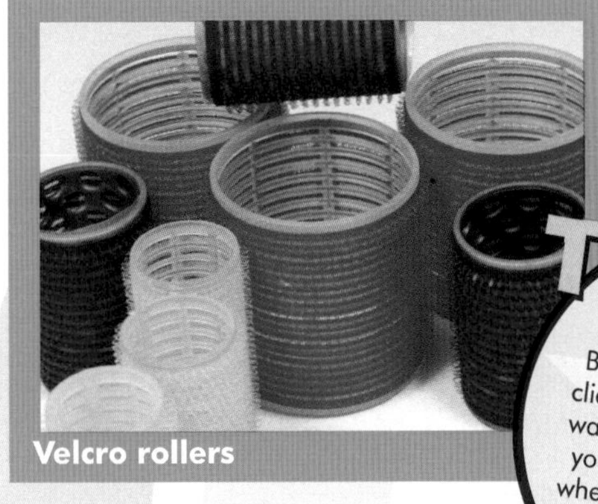
Velcro rollers

TOP TIP

Before shampooing the client's hair, look at which way it goes. This will give you an idea of how and where to place the rollers.

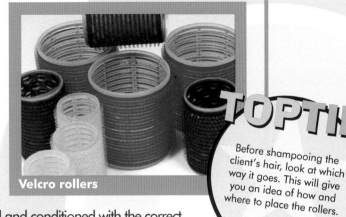

The client's hair must be thoroughly shampooed and conditioned with the correct products for the condition of the client's hair before setting.

How to set hair

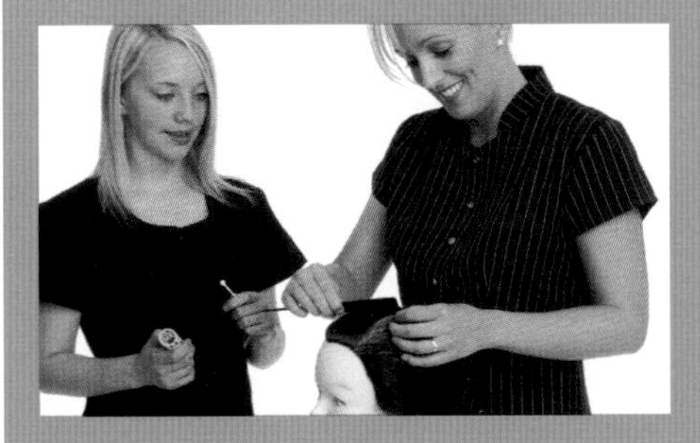

1 Once you have towel dried and disentangled the hair, comb it in the way you will be styling it.

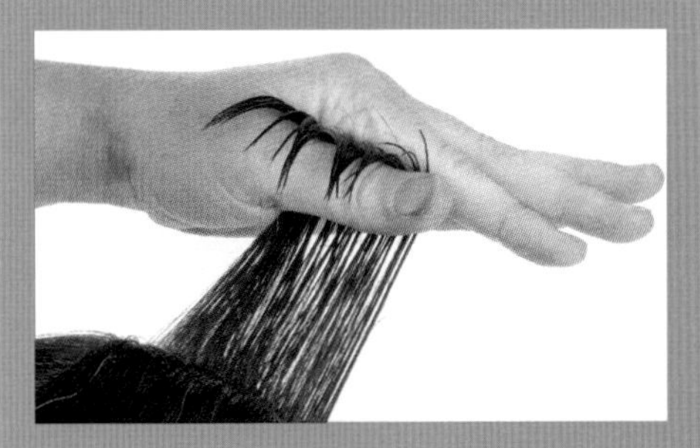

2 Starting at the front hairline, take a section of hair that is the same size as the roller you are going to use. It is important that your sections are really straight.

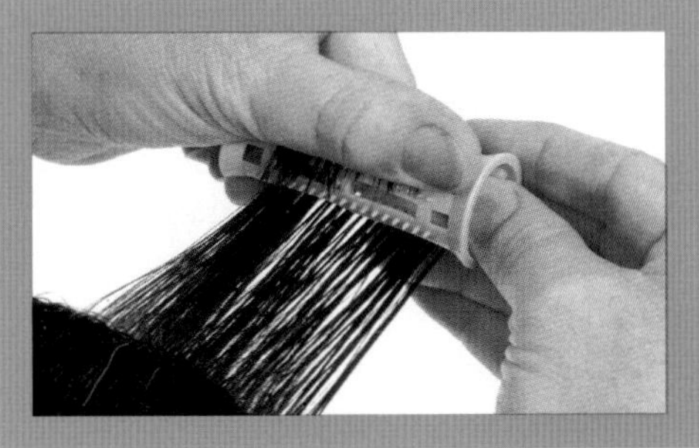

3 Comb the hair so it is really smooth, and then comb it straight up and slightly forward. Put the roller on the ends of the hair, making sure the ends are smooth and tucked around the roller.

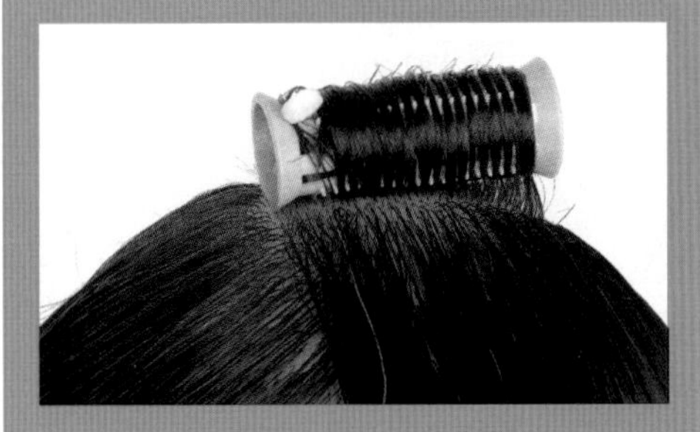

4 Carefully roll down the roller until it sits on the section you took.

It is not good practice to set the hair in straight lines, like a ladder. You will need to learn how to do both brick and directional setting.

TRY IT OUT!

Ask your tutor to demonstrate both brick and directional setting.

Brick setting is done to make sure there are no roller lines showing when you dress out the set. Brick setting looks like the pattern that is made when bricks are laid.

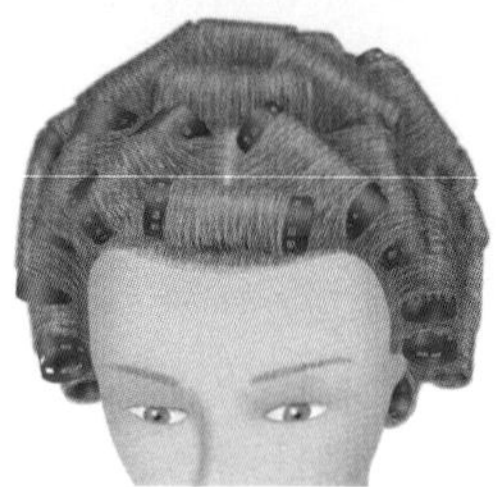

Brick setting looks like the pattern of bricks in a wall

Directional setting is done when a client wants her hair to go in a certain direction, for example if she wants a fringe. It means you have to put the rollers in the way the style will be dressed when it is finished.

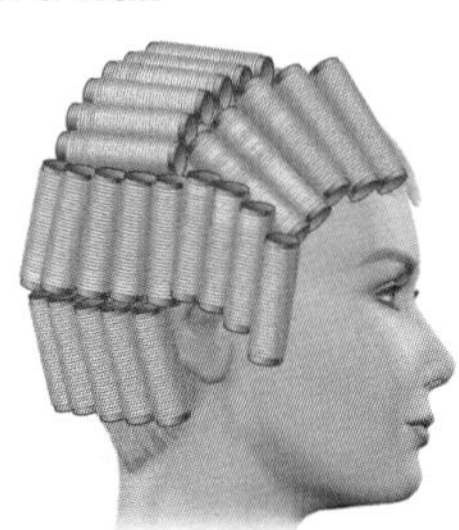

Directional setting

Dressing out the set

This is probably the hardest part of the setting service, as you need to get a really good finish and that takes practice!

When the set comes out from under the hood dryer, you should leave the rollers in the hair while it cools down. This helps to set the hair and make it last longer.

Carefully remove the rollers, then brush the hair using a dressing out brush, starting in the nape and work your way up to the front. The amount of pressure you use when brushing will depend on how thick the client's hair is. However, you must make sure the brush reaches right down to the scalp. This might seem a bit rough but you need to brush the hair firmly to make sure you get rid of any roller lines (and any stiffness in the hair if you have used setting products). Brush the hair up, then down and the way you want the finished style to go. The hair is now ready for you to tease it into the finished style, using a dressing comb.

Your tutor will show you how to tease the hair into its finished style. Once you have finished the dressing out, you should show the client the back of the hair using a hand-held mirror (to make sure she likes it) and then spray with hair spray if needed.

nape: the back of the neck

TOP TIP

As the hair feels hot when it first comes out from the dryer, you may mistakenly think the hair is dry. If the hair is not fully dry, the set will flop. Check a few rollers around the crown area to make sure.

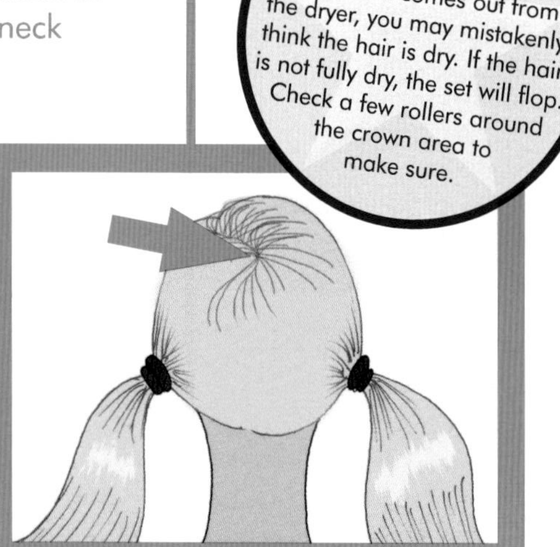

The crown area

Completing the hairdressing service

Once you have finished the hairdressing service, you will need to make sure the client is happy with his or her hair. Clients will be able to see the front of their hair in the mirror, but it is also important to show them the back. The angle you hold the back mirror needs to be just right, otherwise the client will not be able to see.

Dear Nat

I am doing a hairdressing course and am getting really good with my setting and blow-drying. The only problem is, I can't get the hang of where the back mirror should be so the client can see the back of the hair. Can you help?

From Soraya

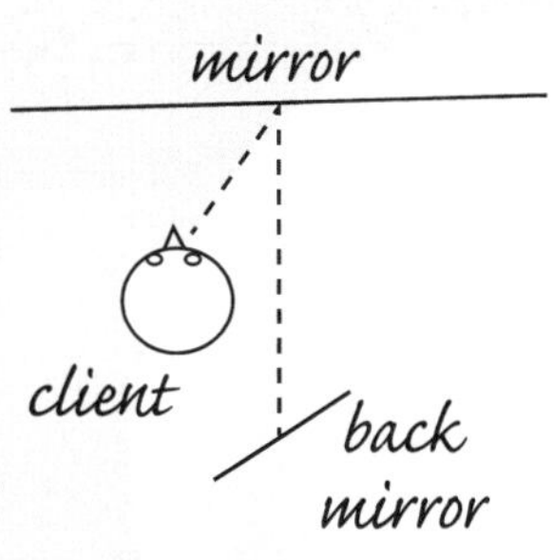

Nat says

Lots of people have problems with the position of the back mirror. I have drawn a diagram showing you where you should be holding the mirror. Both you and the client are looking into the same mirror at the front, so if you can see the back of the hair, it's likely that the client can too!

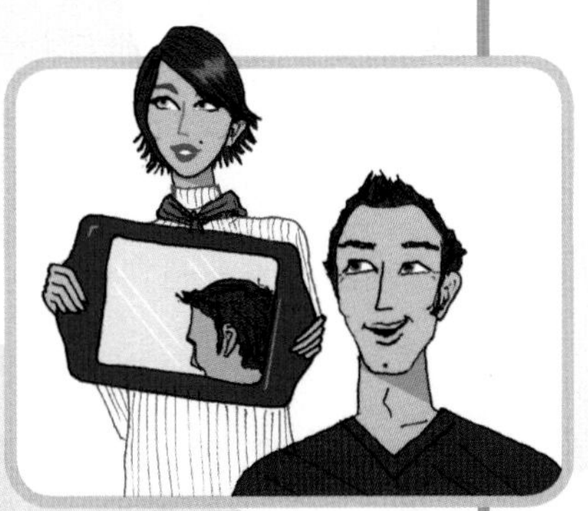

OVER TO YOU...

Find pictures of hair styles that can be achieved with the use of different brushes. They could be from magazines or journals, photographs or sketches. Add them to your portfolio or scrapbook.

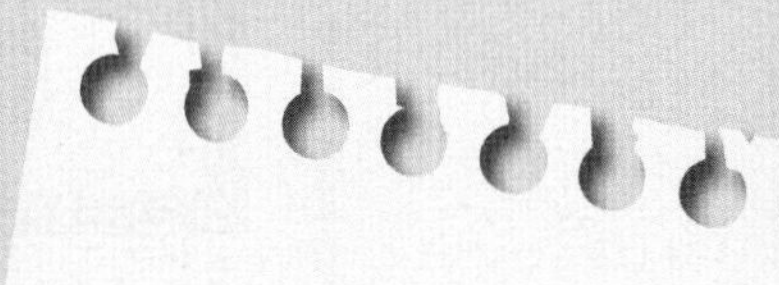

Plaiting and braiding

You can produce some great effects from plaiting and braiding the hair. It can be done 'off scalp', which means the plaits hang loose away from the scalp. Or it can be done 'on scalp', for example French plaits or cane row.

Whether plaiting or braiding on or off the scalp, it is important that you have straight sections, as they are seen when you style the hair. It will look unprofessional if your sections are not straight and even.

How to make a French plait

You will need to prepare the hair before you start plaiting or braiding. It is much easier to plait or braid hair that has not been washed. Newly washed hair tends to be silky soft and difficult to work with.

You may already be able to do some types of plaits and braids, but if not, ask your tutor to show you how to do them.

When the plaits are finished they should be secured using professional bands. These are specially made so they don't damage the hair (as ordinary elastic bands do).

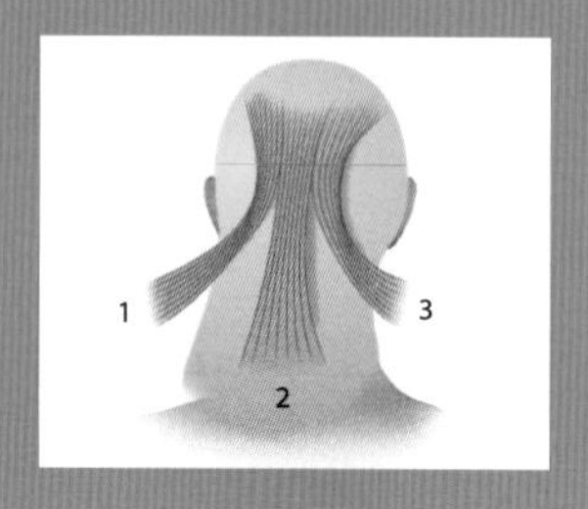

1 Take a small triangle of hair at the front of the head and split into three equal strands.

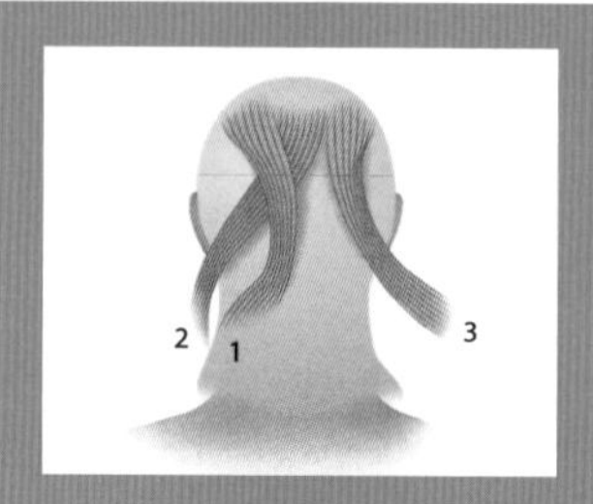

2 Cross the left strand (1) over the centre one (2). The left strand is now the new centre strand.

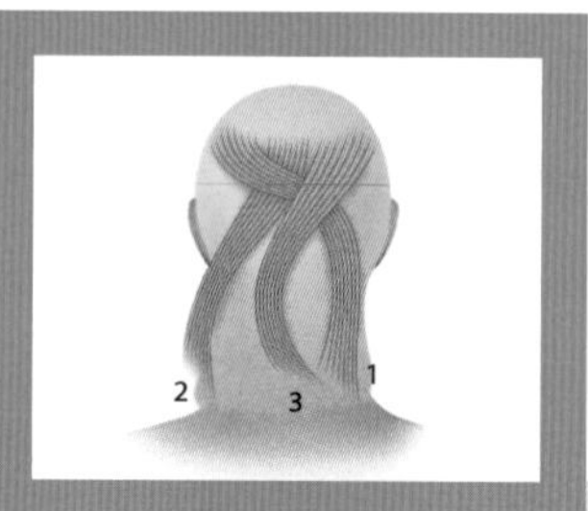

3 Cross the right strand (3) over the centre strand (1). Keep the tension equal in each strand so that the finished braid will be even.

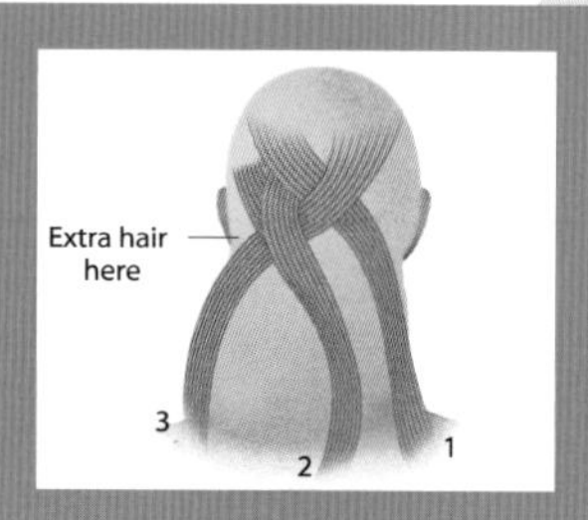

4 Gather extra hair from the left front hairline, about half the thickness of one strand, and add it to the left strand (2). Cross this strand over the centre strand (3).

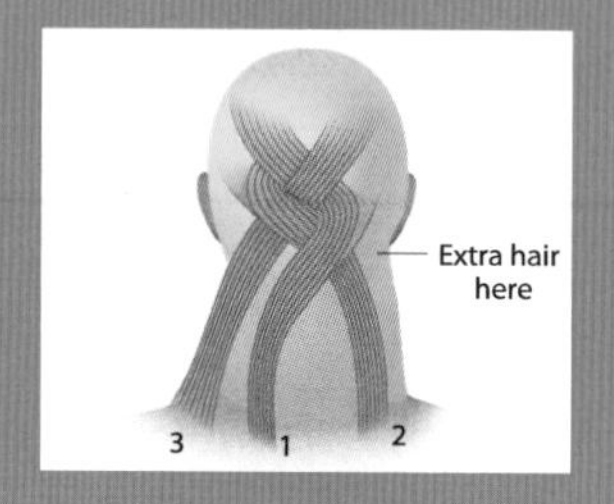

5 Repeat step 4. Add it to the right strand (1) and pass this new strand over the centre strand (2).

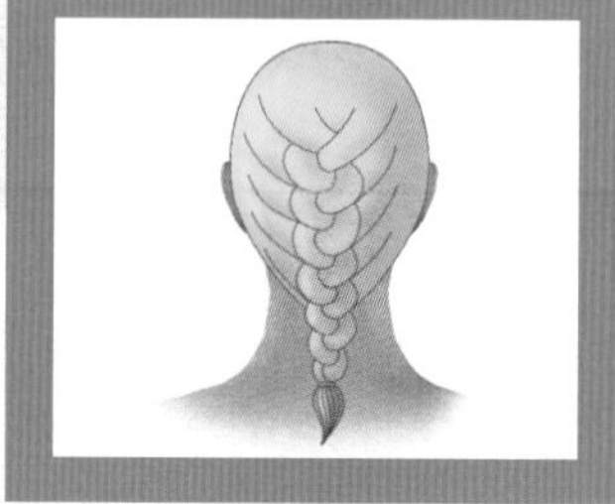

6 Repeat steps 4 and 5 until there is no loose hair at the hairline. Plait the rest of the three strands and secure the ends.

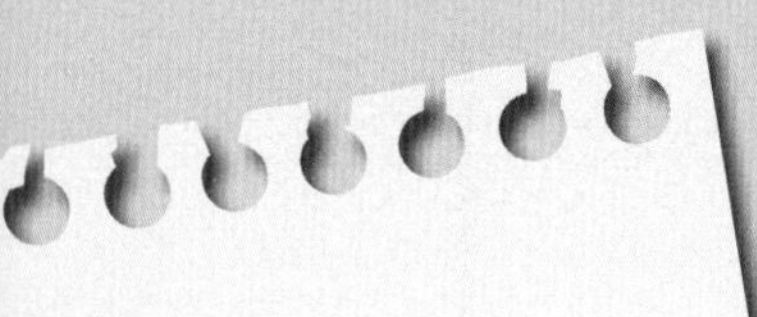

OVER TO YOU...

Find pictures of hair styles that can be achieved with braiding and plaiting. They could be from magazines or journals, photographs or sketches. Add them to your portfolio or scrapbook.

Check what you know...

1. The outside layer of the hair (the bit you can see) is called the:
   - [ ] medulla
   - [ ] cuticle
   - [ ] cortex

2. The shampoo that you would use on greasy hair is:
   - [ ] egg
   - [ ] banana
   - [ ] lemon or lime

3. It is important to gown clients properly to:
   - [ ] protect their clothes from spillages
   - [ ] prevent them from breathing in the hairspray
   - [ ] make sure they are warm throughout the shampooing process

4. Your combs should be sterilised:
   - [ ] in hot soapy water
   - [ ] in a chemical jar
   - [ ] in an autoclave

5. It would be a good idea to use a frontwash if:
   - [ ] your client wears lots of make-up
   - [ ] your client has very long hair
   - [ ] your client has back or neck problems

6. When you are shampooing hair, you should test the temperature of the water on:
   - [ ] the back of your wrist
   - [ ] your upper arm
   - [ ] the client's head

7. The name of the massage movement you use when you are applying shampoo and conditioner is:
   - [ ] petrissage
   - [ ] effleurage
   - [ ] rotary

8. The equipment you should use to secure a plait or braid at the ends is called:
   - [ ] a roller
   - [ ] a butterfly clip
   - [ ] a professional band

9. A brick set would be done to:
   - [ ] make sure the client's hair is curly
   - [ ] make sure the client's hair is straight
   - [ ] prevent roller lines showing when you dress out the set

10. When the set comes out from under the hood dryer, you should leave the rollers in the hair while it cools down as this will:
    - [ ] make sure the client stays in the salon longer
    - [ ] help the hair to set and make it last longer
    - [ ] make it easier to dress out

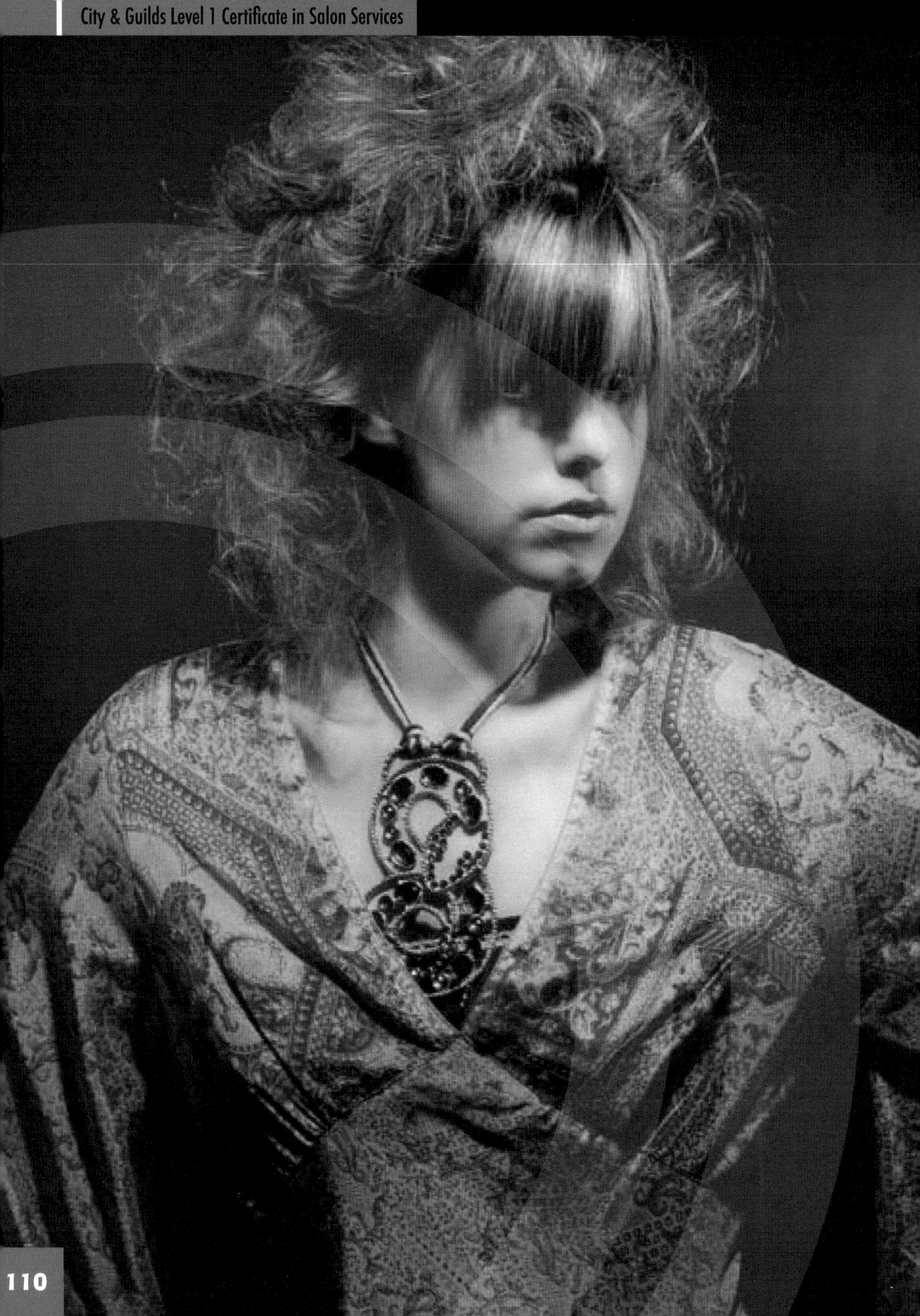

Unit 6

Perming and colouring

This is an important unit because it is all about two of the most exciting services in hairdressing – perming and colouring.

The role you will play in perming and colouring services is a very important one and it is essential that you have had thorough training and are totally committed to the tasks you will be responsible for.

In this unit you will learn about:

- Why we perm hair.
- Why we colour hair.
- Perming and non-permanent colouring equipment.
- The perming and neutralising processes.
- The colouring service.

Towards the end of this unit, you will be observed and assessed on:

- Perming services.
- Colouring hair.

Why we perm hair

Perming is the process of curling the hair permanently using chemicals. Its name comes from the old-fashioned term 'permanent wave'.

Let's look at the reasons for carrying out the perming service:

Reasons for perming
- To add volume and make the hair appear fuller/thicker
- To add a permanent wave or curl to the hair
- To enable the client to maintain a hairstyle at home
- To support the client's chosen hairstyle

Reasons for perming

possibly

Take care when perming and colouring as you are using potentially harmful chemicals. Always follow the manufacturer's instructions and never use products without proper training.

Different styles such as wavy, curly or straight hair go in and out of fashion. In recent years, curly hair has not been especially fashionable and this has resulted in perming being less popular. However, it is still carried out in most salons every day of the week, so it is vital that you fully understand how important it is to get it right.

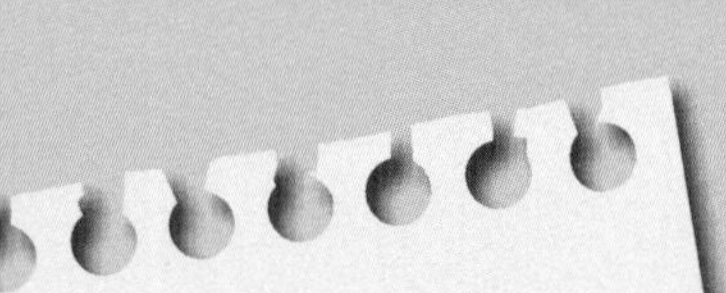

OVER TO YOU...

Find pictures of different looks that have been created using perming techniques. They could be from magazines or journals, photographs or sketches. Show them to a member of staff at the salon where you work or your tutor to check that they really are permed looks. Add them to your portfolio or scrapbook.

Why we colour hair

Below are some of the reasons why a client might come into the salon for a colouring service.

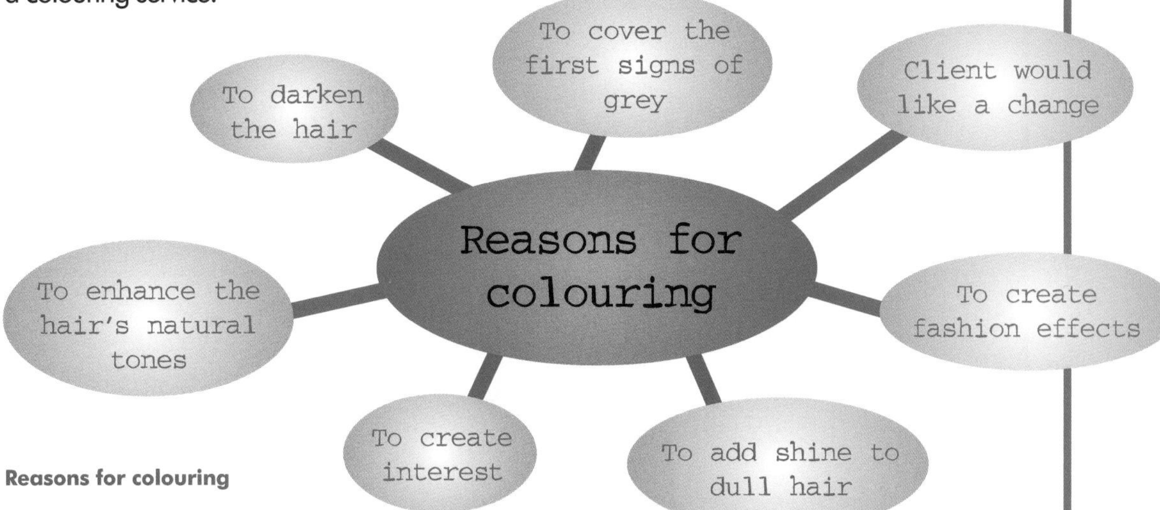
Reasons for colouring
To darken the hair
To cover the first signs of grey
Client would like a change
To enhance the hair's natural tones
To create fashion effects
To create interest
To add shine to dull hair

Reasons for colouring

TRY IT OUT!

Look at the spider diagram above and discuss with salon staff, your tutor or friends why clients might want to add colour to their hair.

You need to consider all the reasons, as this will help you to realise the importance of colouring in the salon.

Perming and non-permanent colouring equipment

Perming and colouring services require a lot of different equipment. Some equipment you will use on yourself and some will be used on the client. You will need to be familiar with each and know how to use it. The essential equipment or 'toolkit' needed for each service is shown on pages 114 and 115. There is also equipment used for client preparation and this is covered further on in this unit.

Equipment used to protect you while perming and colouring is known as **personal protective equipment**, and includes an apron and gloves. These are used to protect your clothes and skin from the harmful chemicals that you will come into contact with and, by law, your employer has to provide them for you to use.

For your own protection, always wear personal protective equipment when carrying out perming and colouring services.

The perming toolkit

Equipment	What it looks like	Uses
Perming rods		These are used to wind the hair in order to fix it into a new shape during the perming process. There are a variety of different lengths, shapes and sizes of rods depending on the curl or wave you want to create.
End papers		These smooth the ends of the hair around the winding rod, to ensure no fish-hook ends.
Sectioning clips		These clip the hair out of the way during winding and developing perms. They come in a variety of different sizes and shapes (you will use the ones that you prefer).
Combs		Various combs are used, e.g. pintail comb for fine sectioning or a wide-tooth comb for detangling.

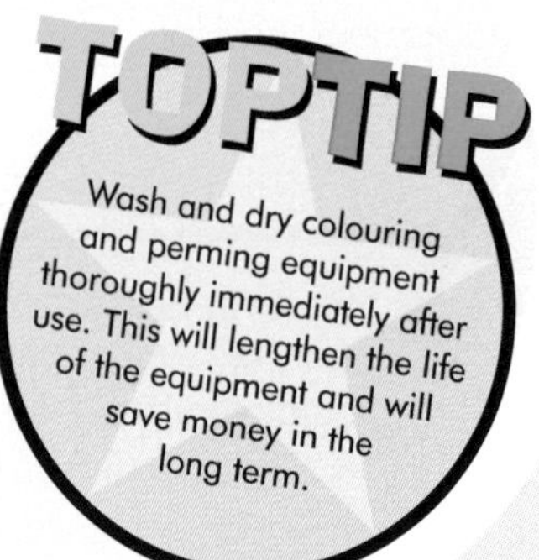

TOPTIP
Wash and dry colouring and perming equipment thoroughly immediately after use. This will lengthen the life of the equipment and will save money in the long term.

The colouring toolkit

Equipment	What it looks like	Uses
Colour mixing bowl		This is used to mix colours in. There should be one for each separate colour used. It is a good idea to either label or colour coordinate when using more than one colour, e.g. if using a red and blonde use a red and a white bowl.
Combs		Various combs are used, e.g. a pintail comb for fine weaving or a wide tooth comb for detangling.
Tinting brushes /sponges (only tinting brush shown here)		Both are used to apply colour but in different ways. A sponge is used to colour large areas. A tinting brush allows the colour to be applied more accurately to a specific area.
Applicator bottle		This is used to apply colour directly to the hair. The bottle usually has a long, thin nozzle that allows you to section the hair ready for application.
Sectioning clips		These clip the hair out of the way while colouring. They come in a variety of different sizes and shapes (you will use the ones that you prefer).

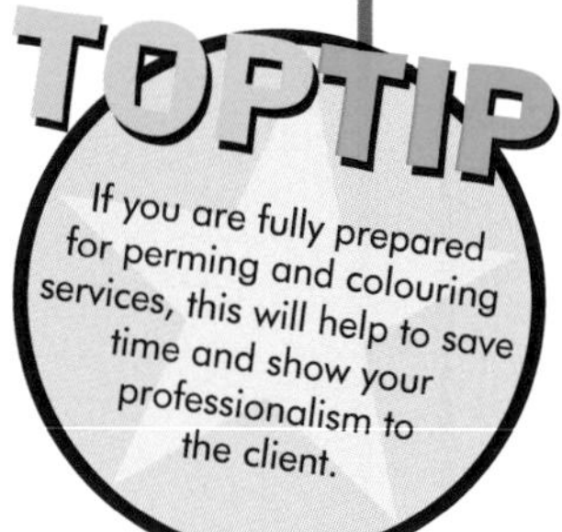
TOPTIP
If you are fully prepared for perming and colouring services, this will help to save time and show your professionalism to the client.

Preparing the client

As the salon junior, it is likely you will be responsible for preparing clients for perming and colouring services. Look at the client preparation toolkit below. Learn each of the items and their uses, as they are very important for client preparation and comfort during colouring and perming services. Don't worry, you won't be expected to prepare a client until you have been shown the correct way by the staff at the salon.

Always ask the client if he or she is comfortable with the protection provided both before the service begins and throughout.

Client preparation toolkit

Equipment	What it looks like	Uses
Gowns		These protect the client's clothing from spillages and drips.
Towels		These are placed around the client's neck (over the gown) to protect from spillages and drips.
Tissues and cotton wool		These are used around the hairline or neckline to protect the client's skin from coming into contact with the chemicals used.

The photo shows a client who has been well prepared for perming and colouring services. Your salon may use a different type of gown or even plastic shoulder capes, but the main priority is that the client is adequately protected and comfortable both before and during the service.

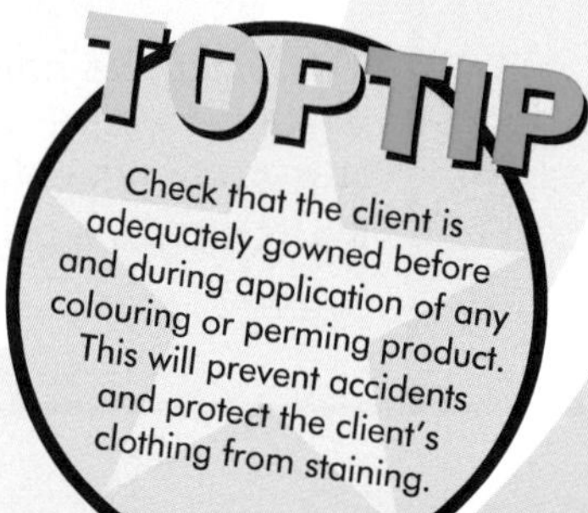
TOPTIP
Check that the client is adequately gowned before and during application of any colouring or perming product. This will prevent accidents and protect the client's clothing from staining.

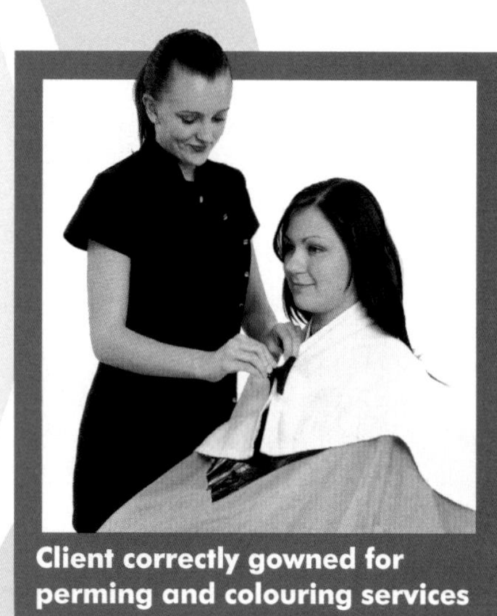
Client correctly gowned for perming and colouring services

Dear Nat

Last week, I had to get a client ready for a colouring service for one of the senior stylists. I put the gown on and a towel around her shoulders and left her for the stylist, but when the service was finished the client had some colour on her top. She complained to the salon and has asked them to pay for cleaning or a replacement. The stylist tried to blame me. She said that as I had gowned the client, it was my responsibility. I don't agree with her as I didn't apply the colour and so I can't have got it on her clothes. What should I do now?

From Jo

Nat says

You are right in that the stylist is responsible for making sure that the client is properly protected during application and development of any colour service that he or she carries out. You will need to stick up for yourself here and speak to your boss about it. However, since you initially gowned the client, you will have to accept some responsibility and apologise. You have learned a valuable lesson here – how easy it is to let standards slip and what the consequences can be, but also to be professional and accept responsibility and apologise for the things you have done wrong.

Keeping the work area clean and tidy

Before, during and after a perming or a colouring service you must maintain and clean the work area:

- Before the service, check the work area is clean and tidy and set up the correct equipment – this shows professionalism and will send a message to the client that he or she can have confidence in your ability.
- During the service, check the work area for used towels and tint bowls and any used consumables such as end papers or cotton wool that can be removed and cleared away – this will show the client that you are keeping the work area clean and tidy and again looks professional.
- After the service, when the client has moved away from the area, put away equipment, wipe over the trolley (if used) and dispose of any unused products in line with your salon's policy – this will ensure that the work area is clean, ready for the next client.

consumables: items that are used once and then thrown away

The perming and neutralising processes

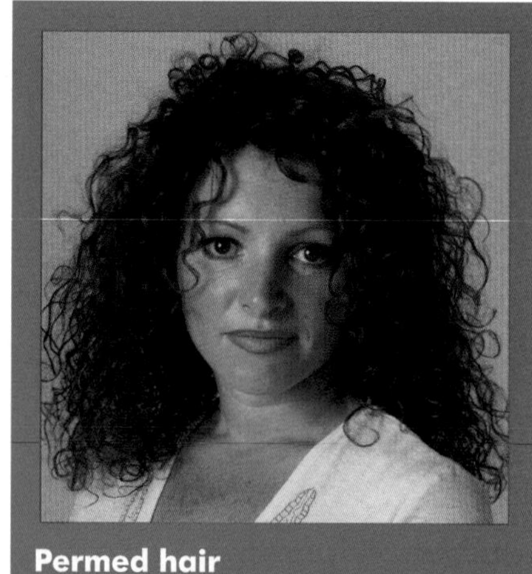

Permed hair

Winding the perm

Winding the perm is the part of the perming process where small, neat and even sections of the hair are taken and wrapped around perm rods, using the correct amount of tension.

stretch, tightness

Before you begin the perm wind, you should divide the hair into neat and even sections and ensure it is tangle free. This will allow you to wind the hair in a methodical pattern and will help to keep the tension even on the wind. Below is an illustration of how the hair should be divided into nine sections ready for the perm wind to begin.

step-by-step

Each time you wind a mesh of hair, take care with the placing of the end paper to avoid fish hooks.

a small section of hair

hair ends buckled or bent during winding

Ensure that each mesh you section off is even and neat to prevent root drag which causes the client discomfort and damages the hair.

Make sure that the rod is wound correctly on the base, again to prevent root drag.

Take care when fastening each rod that you don't twist the rubber or fasten too tightly as this can cause the client discomfort and damages the hair.

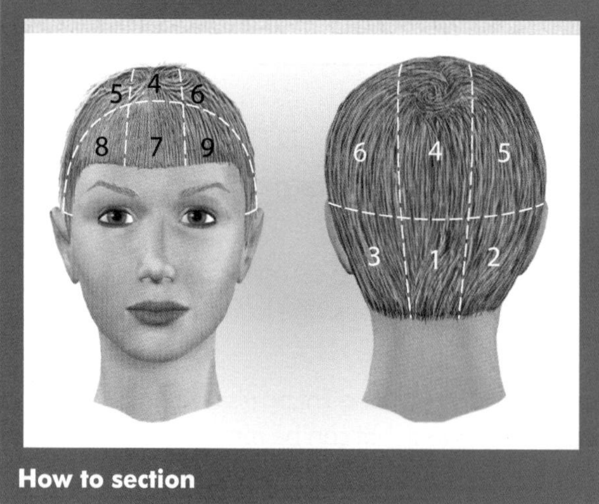

How to section

How to perm wind a client's hair

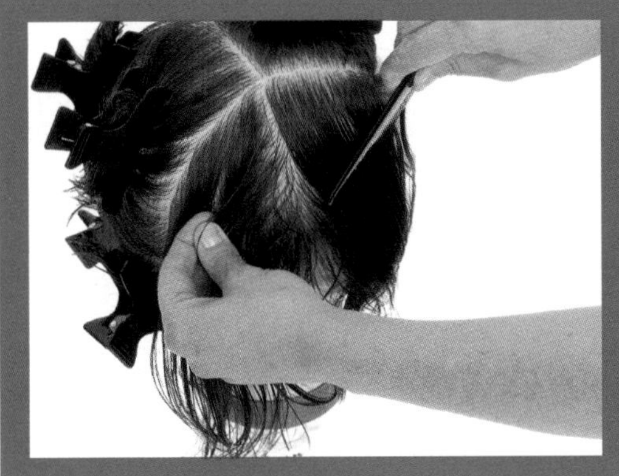

1 Divide the hair into neat and even sections.

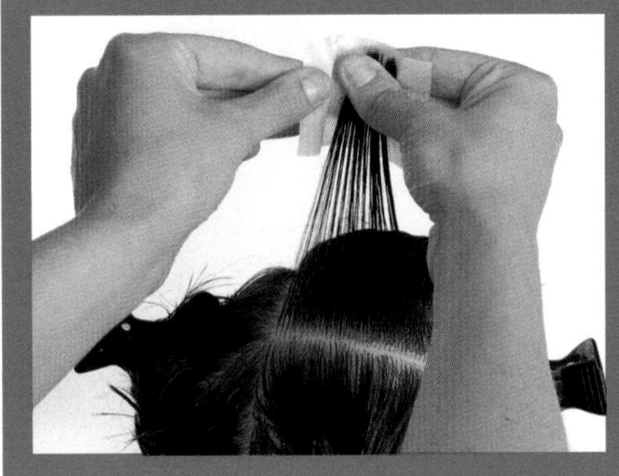

2 Place the end paper carefully around the hair ends.

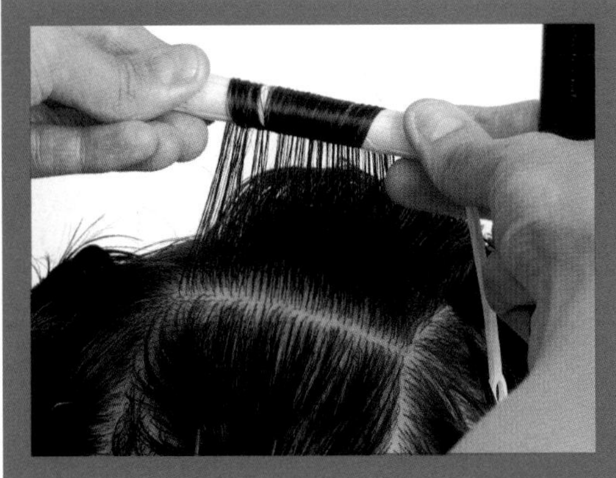

3 Wind the hair using the perm rod from the ends down to the root.

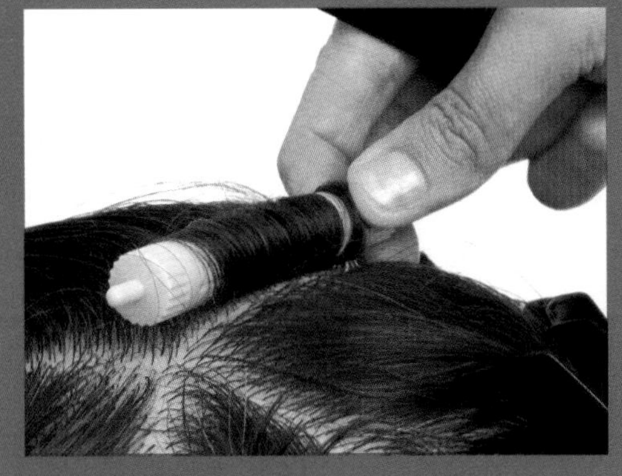

4 Place the rod correctly on the base. Ensure that you wind the hair so that it sits on the base of the mesh you have wound it from.

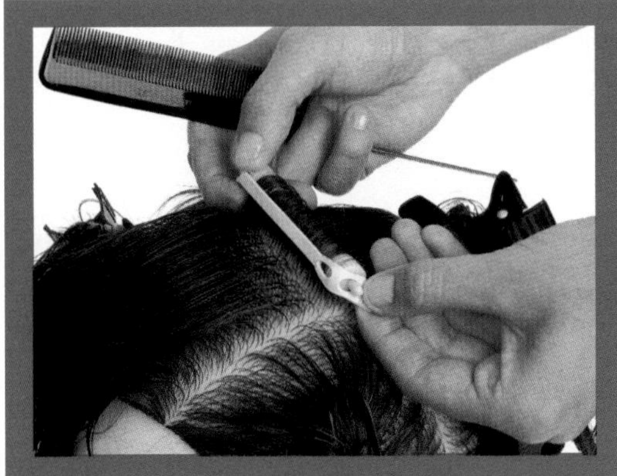

5 Fasten the rod correctly. Take care to fasten the rubber without twisting and with enough tension to hold the rod in place but without pulling the hair too tightly.

Dear Nat

I am getting very frustrated with my perm winding, I just can't do it! Each time I manage to get the rods in most of them are too loose or have fish-hook ends. What am I doing wrong? Why can't I do it like the stylists in the salon?

From Jenna

Nat says

First, don't get upset. Look at all the experience the staff in your salon have had of winding perms – I bet they've been doing it for years! Secondly, remember that you have only just started your training and it really does take time and lots of practice to get it right. No one said hairdressing would be easy, but if you just show commitment and belief in your ability, then it will all fall into place. Next time, ask your tutor or a staff member to watch you carefully while you wind a perm and correct you as you go along. This will point out any errors you are making and they can suggest how you can put them right. Good luck and keep trying!

Neutralising the perm

often

Neutralising is the second stage of the perming process and takes place only once the perm has developed fully. This is a process that most salon juniors carry out frequently and usually takes place at the basin area as it involves rinsing and applying lotions.

During neutralising, the curl that you have made by winding the hair around the rod and then applying perm lotion now becomes fixed into its new shape. (Chemical changes have taken place inside the hair structure that make the curl stay permanently.) Neutralising is a very important part of the perming process. If neutralising is not carried out correctly, the perm will not be successful.

Always check with a senior member of staff that you are using the correct neutraliser for the perm that has been used before beginning the neutralising process. This will ensure a good curl result and the hair will not be chemically damaged.

The neutralising process

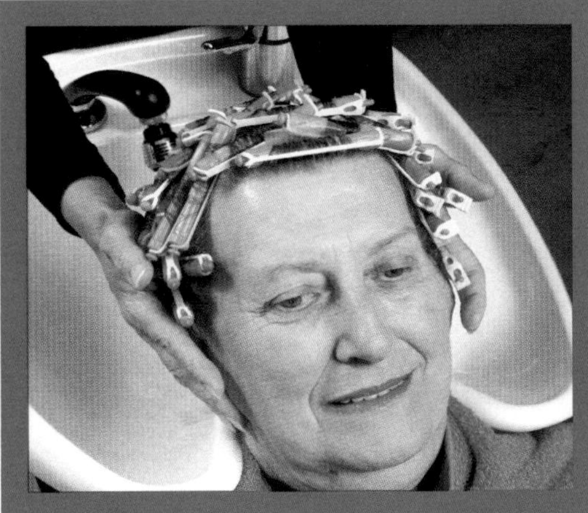

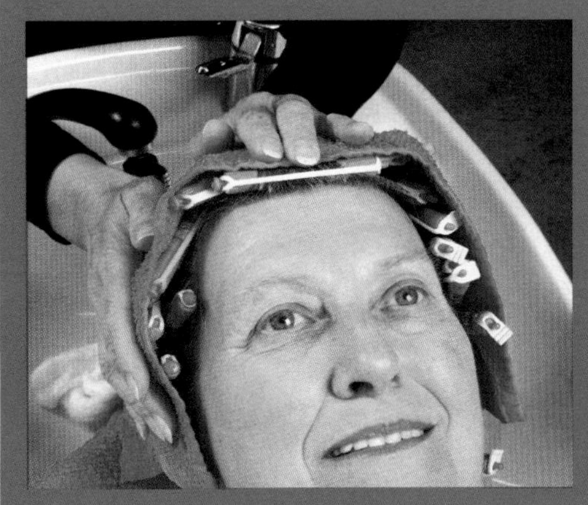

1 Thoroughly rinse the hair to remove all the perm lotion. Remember to check the water temperature is comfortable with the client as the scalp may be sensitive following the perm development. It is important to keep the flow of water constant and direct the water away from the client's face all the way through rinsing.

2 Once the hair has been thoroughly rinsed for the recommended time, remove excess water from the hair by blotting with a dry towel, cotton wool or tissue.

more than is needed

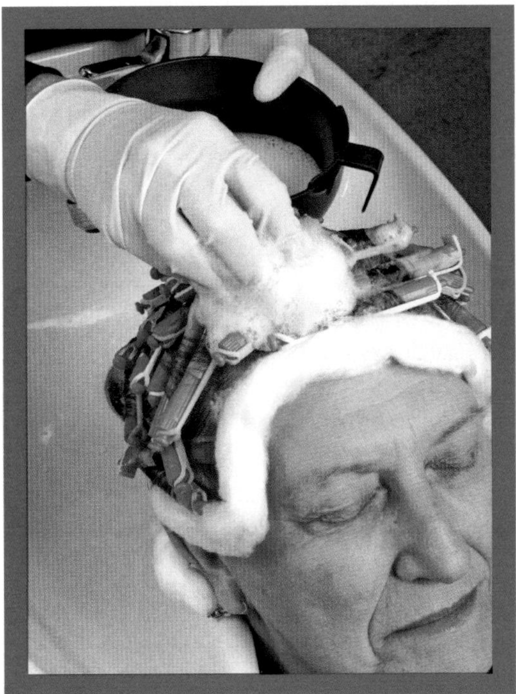

3 Use cotton wool around the client's hairline to protect from drips onto the face or neck. Prepare and apply the neutraliser as shown in the manufacturer's instructions. Follow these instructions carefully to ensure a good result. You must use the correct neutraliser for the type of perm solution that has been used. If not, you could cause chemical damage to the hair and you risk a poor result.

4 Leave the neutraliser on the hair for the stated time (check the manufacturer's instructions). Too short a time may result in a poor curl. Too long may result in chemical damage.

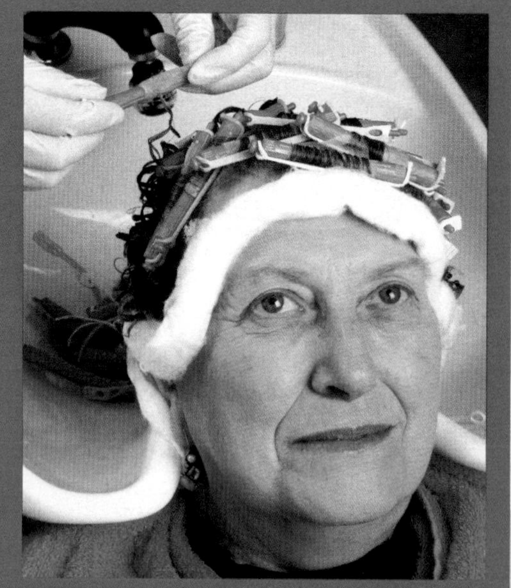

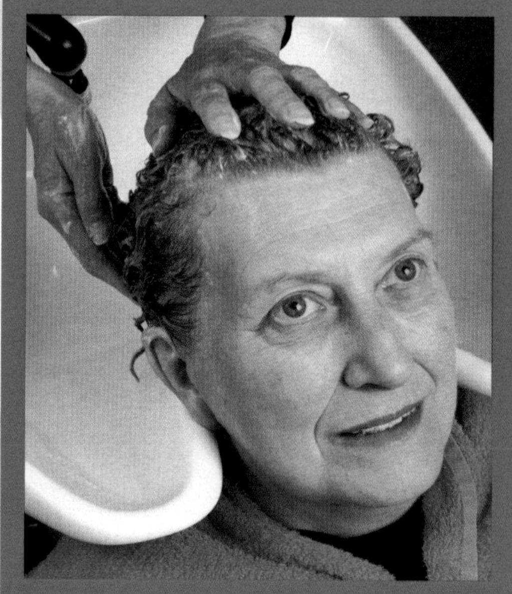

5 Once the hair has been developed with neutraliser for the correct time, carefully remove the rods. Don't drag or pull the hair, which will cause the client discomfort and risk damaging the hair. Once all the perm rods have been removed, rinse the neutraliser from the hair. Again, check the water temperature and direct away from the face, keeping the flow constant. Read the manufacturer's recommended rinse time, but ensure the hair is thoroughly rinsed.

6 Apply a suitable conditioner. If the product does not provide one with the perm lotion and neutraliser, then it is recommended to use an anti-oxidant conditioner. This will stop the chemicals you have used in the neutraliser from working and help to smooth the hair and leave it soft and manageable.

Throughout the neutralising process check your client's comfort. Ask the client if he or she is well protected and dry. Also check that the scalp is not irritated by any of the chemicals you are using.

Congratulations, you have successfully completed the neutralising process! You can return the client to the stylist ready for further styling.

salon scene

A client returns for her regular blow-dry one week after having her hair permed at the salon. When you have finished shampooing and conditioning the hair and are de-tangling it you notice that the hair appears to be straight at the back throughout the nape area. You tell the client immediately that you think her perm has fallen out at the back and she becomes quite upset and asks for the manager. The manager comes across immediately and explains to the client that the perm looks to have 'dropped' considerably in a small area but that it can be re-permed without difficulty straightaway and it will only take about 40 minutes to complete. The client seems much calmer now and is happy to go ahead with the re-perm.

When the client has left the salon your manager tells you off, saying that you should not have mentioned anything to the client but informed him **discreetly** straightaway. He blames you, saying that you obviously didn't neutralise the hair thoroughly the week before.

discreetly: quietly and secretively without causing a fuss

Are you solely responsible for the under-neutralising of this perm?

Why do you think the manager was angry with you for telling the client her perm had fallen out?

The colouring service

As with perming, and indeed all hairdressing services, there are fashion trends within colouring. In recent years, there have been exciting developments in non-permanent colouring. These include glitter gels and sprays and hair mascara in bright fashion shades that are brushed onto the hair directly from the bottle.

Look back to the beginning of the unit to remind yourself why clients might want a colour service.

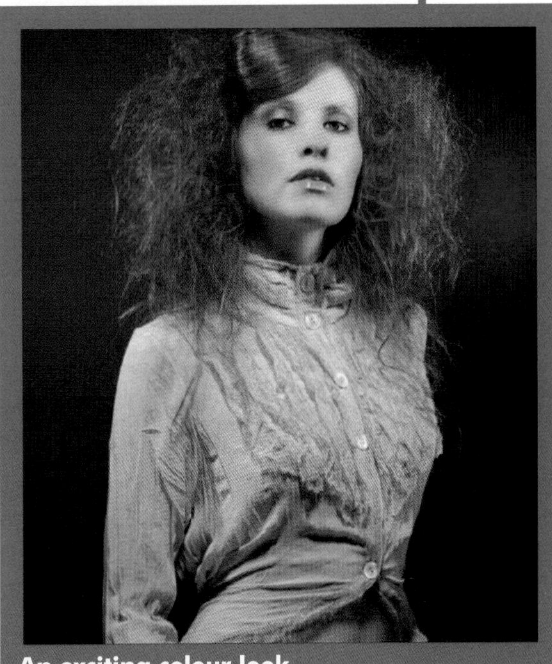
An exciting colour look

Temporary and semi-permanent colours

Temporary and semi-permanent colours are known as non-permanent colouring. This means the colours do not last and will shampoo out of the hair rather than grow out. The table below gives you some information on why we use temporary and semi-permanent colours.

Type of colour	Effect on hair structure	Uses	How long the colour lasts
Temporary	Temporary colour molecules are large and coat the cuticle	Enhances the natural hair colour by adding tones Darkens natural or coloured hair but will not make hair appear lighter Can be used to create fashion effects	1 shampoo – only puts colour onto the outer layer of the hair (cuticle)
Semi-permanent	Semi-permanent colour molecules are large and small. Large molecules coat the cuticle and small molecules enter the cortex	Enhances the natural hair colour by adding tones Darkens natural or coloured hair but will not make hair appear lighter Can be used to create fashion effects	4 – 8 shampoos If the hair is porous, the cutical scales will be lifted and colour can make its way just inside the cortex.

a very small particle of colour that can only be seen under a micro-scope

make more noticeable

lets liquid through

OVER TO YOU...

Find pictures of hair that looks coloured using both temporary and semi-permanent colours. They could be from magazines or journals, photographs or sketches. Show them to a member of staff at the salon or your tutor to see if they really are the coloured looks you are looking for. Add them to your portfolio or scrapbook.

Establishing a client's colouring requirements

You will need to carry out a colouring consultation in order to establish what the client wants. Here is an example of a colouring consultation form that would be used in a salon. Of course, it covers permanent colouring also, so some of the information such as peroxide strengths would not be relevant to a non-permanent colour service.

find out

Colouring Consultation Form

Client's name ______

Address ______

Post code ______ Contact tel no ______

Colouring: Base shade ______ Tones ______

Amount of white hair present:
☐ 0–10% ☐ 10–25% ☐ 25–50% ☐ 50–75% ☐ 75–100%

Colourant type:
☐ Temporary ☐ Semi-permanent ☐ Quasi-permanent ☐ Permanent
☐ Bleach ☐ Lightening ☐ Darkening ☐ Changing tone

Product chosen:
Name ______ Shade no ______
With/without heat ______ Processing time ______

Peroxide strength:
☐ 10 vol (3%) ☐ 20 vol (6%) ☐ 30 vol (9%) ☐ 40 vol (12%)

Method of application:
☐ Full head ☐ Re-growth ☐ High/lowlights ☐ Foils ☐ Mesh ☐ Other

Colour result and evaluation ______

After-care advice ______

A colour consultation form

You need to ask the client questions in order to build a picture of exactly what the client needs and whether or not you can carry out the service. Don't worry too much at this stage, as you will be supported in this type of activity until you feel confident enough to complete it on your own. Even then, until you are fully qualified, you should always check the client's requirements and your suggestions for colouring with a senior member of staff.

Preparing for the colour service

You will have to follow a routine before you begin to apply colour to the client's hair and this involves several stages of preparation:

method or procedure

- Choose an application method – to ensure the product is applied correctly.
- Choose suitable equipment for the desired result and prepare the work area – this saves time and looks professional.
- Prepare the client's hair for the chosen technique – to ensure the colour is applied appropriately.
- Prepare the colour product in accordance with the

Always follow the manufacturer's instructions when preparing a colour product as this is an essential health and safety requirement.

Until you feel confident carrying out all of the above tasks you will be supported in your activities by the salon staff or your tutor. Eventually with a little experience you will be able to prepare on your own without help.

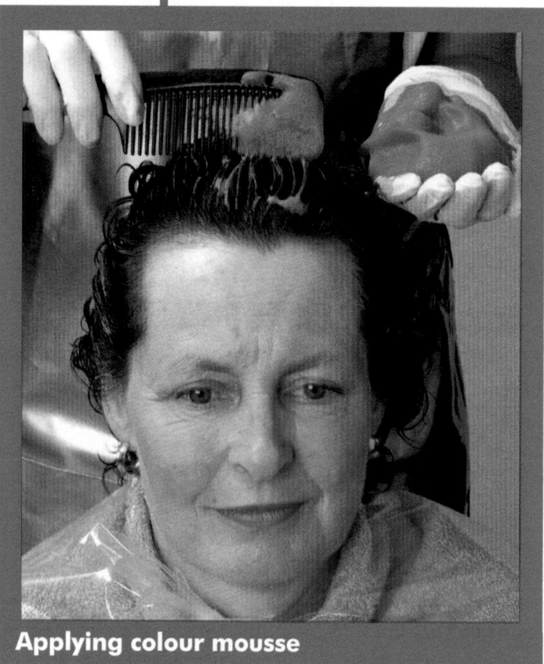

Applying colour mousse

Applying non-permanent colour

Non-permanent colour can be applied to the hair in a variety of ways. It is best to carefully read and follow the manufacturer's instructions supplied with each product. The two main methods are:

- The wet (damp) method – where the hair is shampooed and towel dried before application.
- The dry method – where the colour is applied directly to dry hair.

Look at the tables which list the different types of temporary and semi-permanent colours and how to apply them to the hair.

Always use the appropriate personal protective equipment when carrying out a colour service to ensure that your skin does not come into contact with the chemicals which can cause dermatitis.

How to apply semi-permanent colours

Type of colour	Application method	Application technique
Cream	Apply to damp hair	Section the hair and apply either by massaging into the hair using a tint bowl and brush or a tint bowl and sponge. Take care not to stain the scalp.
Mousse	Apply to damp hair	Section the hair and apply either by massaging or combing into the hair. Take care not to stain the scalp.
Liquid	Apply to damp hair	Section the hair and apply either directly from the bottle using the applicator nozzle provided or use a tint bowl and brush or a tint bowl and sponge. Take care not to stain the scalp.

How to apply temporary colours

Type of colour	Application method	Application technique
Setting lotions	Apply to damp hair	Can be applied directly from the bottle and sprinkled onto the hair and massaged in. Take care not to stain the scalp.
Gels	Apply to either dry or damp hair	Can be applied directly from the bottle either with fingers (using gloves) or with an applicator provided. Take care not to overload the hair with product.
Mousses	Apply to damp hair	Massage or comb into the hair. Take care not to overload the hair with product or stain the scalp.
Water rinses	Apply to damp hair	Rinse through the hair at the backwash using the bottle provided.
Hair spray	Apply to dry hair	Spray directly onto the hair as required. Take care not to stain the scalp and cover hair that is not to be coloured before spraying.
Glitter spray	Apply to dry hair	Spray directly onto the hair as required and cover hair that is not to be coloured.
Colour paints	Apply to dry hair	Apply using the nozzle provided or with fingers. Take care not to overload the hair with product.

The four golden rules

When applying colour to hair always follow these four golden rules:

1. Make neat and even partings when sectioning the hair to ensure the product is applied evenly throughout the hair.
2. Ensure you apply enough of the colour product but do not overload the hair.
3. Take care when monitoring the development time. Leave to develop for the specified time according to the manufacturer's instructions to ensure good coverage.
4. Always remove excess colour product immediately to prevent staining of the skin or scalp.

Applying temporary colours

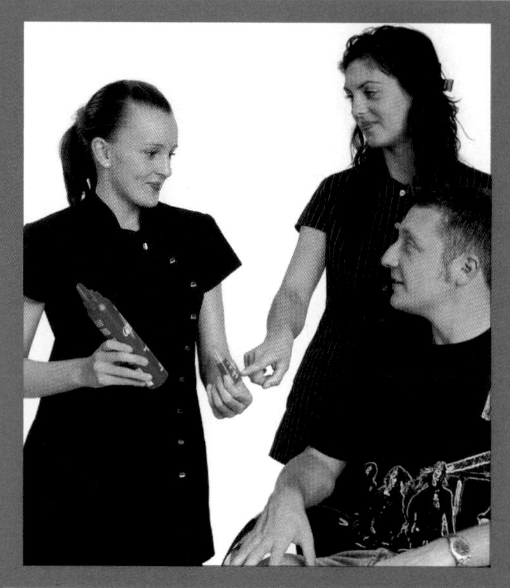

1 Select the colour with the client.

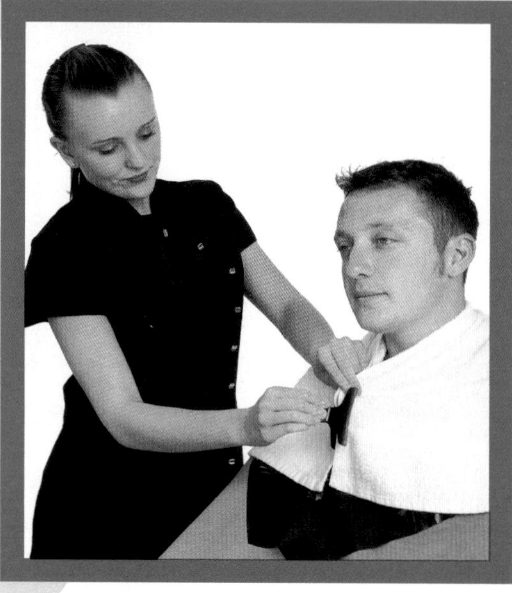

2 Gown and protect the client.

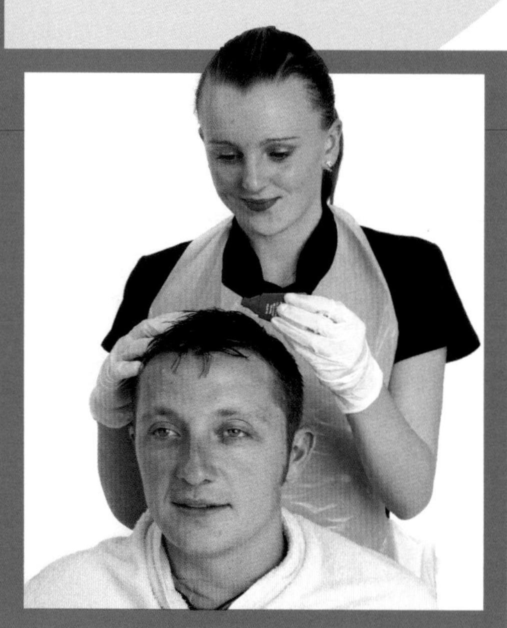

3 Apply the colour. A setting lotion is being applied here.

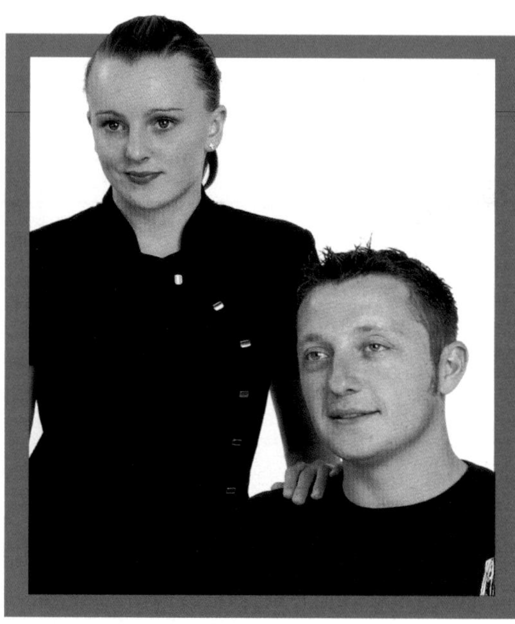

4 The finished effect

Applying semi-permanent colours

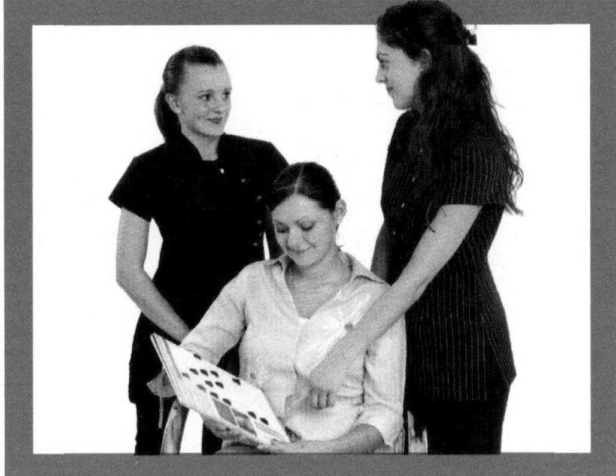

1 Select the colour with the client.

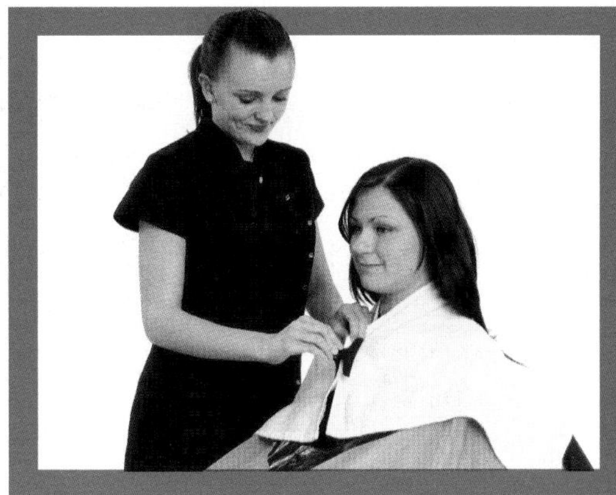

2 Gown and protect the client.

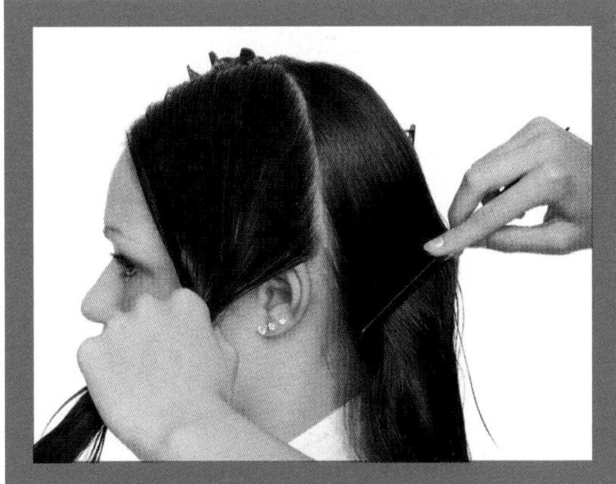

3 Section the hair.

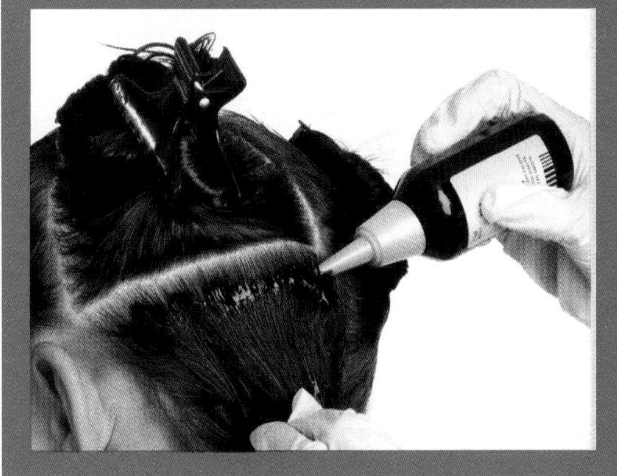

4 Apply the colour. A liquid colour is being applied here.

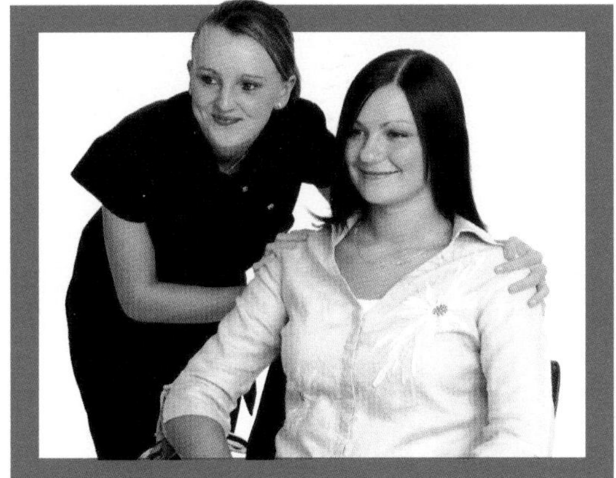

5 The finished effect.

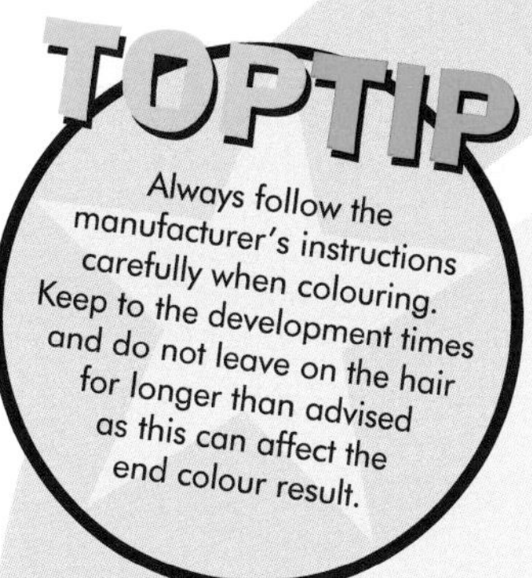

TOP TIP

Always follow the manufacturer's instructions carefully when colouring. Keep to the development times and do not leave on the hair for longer than advised as this can affect the end colour result.

salon scene

A client returns to the salon to complain about a stained collar on her blouse following a colouring service. While you were taking her gown at reception you had noticed that she had colour on the collar but did not want to upset her, so decided to say nothing. Your boss deals with the situation by apologising and offering to have the blouse cleaned to remove the stain. Since your boss accepted responsibility for the stain, the client felt satisfied.

What should you have done when you spotted the staining?

What might have happened to the salon's reputation if the client had not returned to complain but had told other people about what had happened?

Should you now tell your boss about your error of judgement and that you have learned from it?

Check what you know...

Watch out! Some questions have more than one correct answer.

1. Why must you always gown and protect a client thoroughly before a perming or colouring service?
   - [ ] to ensure the client is adequately protected from chemicals
   - [ ] it looks professional
   - [ ] to spend more time pampering the client
2. Why should you always prepare the work area ready for a perming or colouring service?
   - [ ] to prevent you using the wrong tool
   - [ ] to save time and it looks professional
   - [ ] so that the client can see what you are using
3. Why must you section the hair prior to winding a perm?
   - [ ] to waste time
   - [ ] to allow you to work neatly and methodically
   - [ ] to ensure you take the right size sections
4. Why should end papers be used when perming?
   - [ ] it looks good
   - [ ] to stop the perm lotion going on the ends of the hair
   - [ ] to ensure the ends of the hair are smoothly wrapped around the perm rod
5. Why do you need to monitor the neutralising development time accurately?
   - [ ] to be sure that the neutraliser has fixed the curl in place
   - [ ] to prevent under neutralising and the curl dropping out
   - [ ] to make sure the perm rods do not dissolve
6. When should you put away the tools and equipment following service?
   - [ ] before you have finished to keep tidy
   - [ ] when you have finished with something
   - [ ] at the end of the day in case you need them again
7. Why might you need to section the hair before applying colour?
   - [ ] to ensure that the colour is applied evenly to all of the hair
   - [ ] so that the client will feel comfortable
   - [ ] so that you can work methodically and professionally
8. Why should you always follow the manufacturer's instructions carefully?
   - [ ] in case you need to wash the perm or colour off the hair early
   - [ ] to prevent any mistakes in the perming or colouring process
   - [ ] it is breaking the law if you don't
9. Should you be advising clients about the colour for their hair without supervision?
   - [ ] yes, this is not a problem
   - [ ] only if you feel confident
   - [ ] no, even if you feel confident you should always check with someone with more experience than you
10. Why should you use a client consultation sheet when perming or colouring?
    - [ ] to keep busy
    - [ ] to keep a written record of what has been said
    - [ ] to prevent any misunderstandings between the client's requirements and what you think the client has said

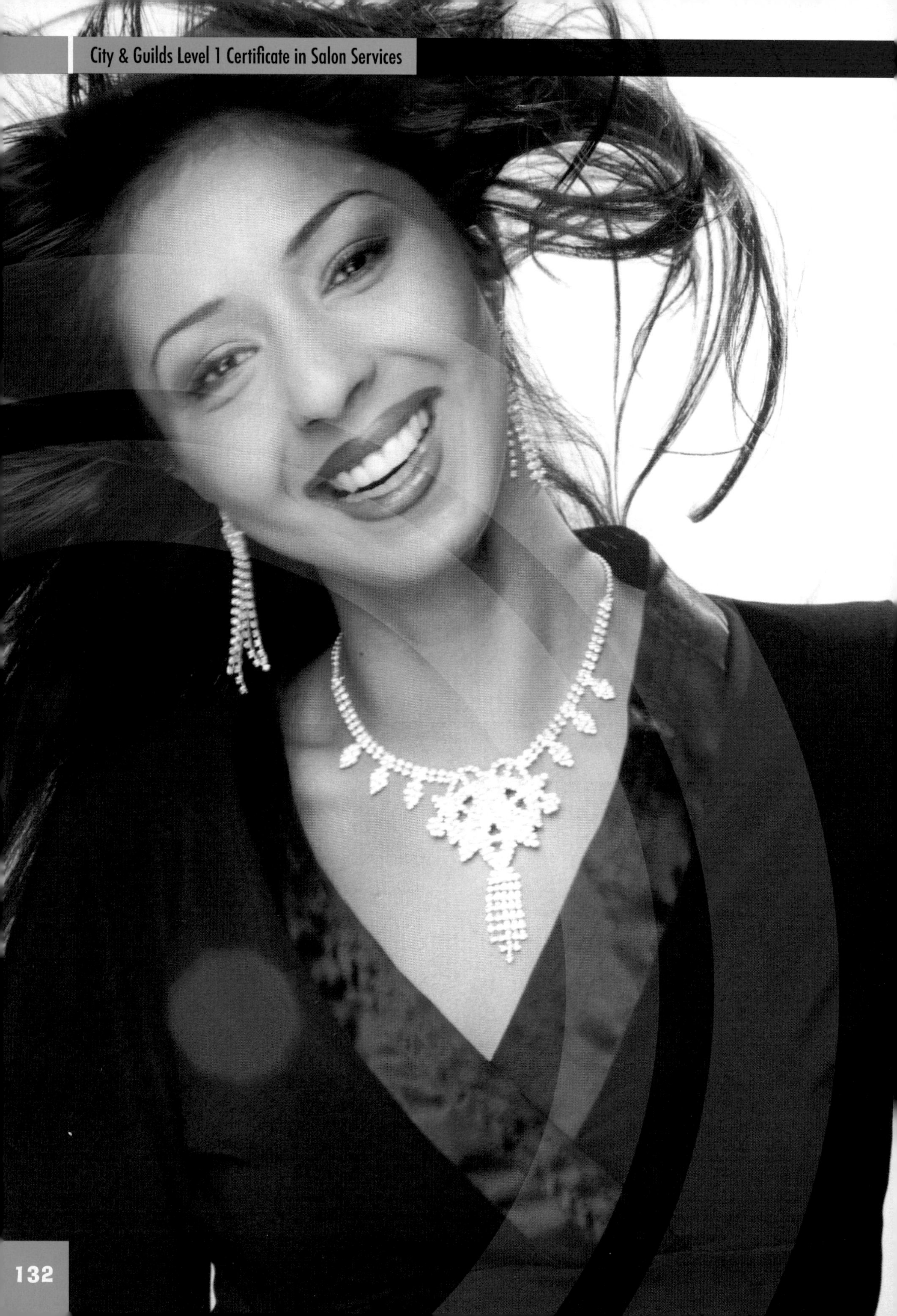

Unit 7

Basic make-up

You have probably only ever applied your own make-up or that of friends using products from your cosmetic bag. But the art of professional make-up application gives a great sense of satisfaction to both the client and artist. From the use of dazzling colours and creative methods to technical know-how, make-up application is a skill that can be learned whatever your artistic ability.

In this unit you will learn about:

- The structure and functions of the skin.
- Why we apply make-up.
- Skin types, conditions, disorders and reactions.
- Products, materials and equipment for make-up treatments.
- Applying make-up products.

Towards the end of the course, you will be observed and assessed on:

- Setting up your work area.
- Carrying out a basic make-up.
- Tidying up after the treatment.

The structure and functions of the skin

The skin's structure

The skin has three main layers:

- The epidermis – the surface layer.
- The dermis – the deeper layer.
- The subcutaneous or fatty layer.

The epidermis

This is the outermost layer of the skin. It is thickest on the soles of the feet and the palms of the hand, and thinnest on the eyelids. The thickness of the epidermis also varies with skin type.

The dermis

The dermis lies just below the epidermis. It contains the skin's blood supply, nerve endings, sweat glands, oil glands and hair muscles.

The subcutaneous layer

This lies below the dermis and gives warmth and protection to the muscles, bones and internal organs.

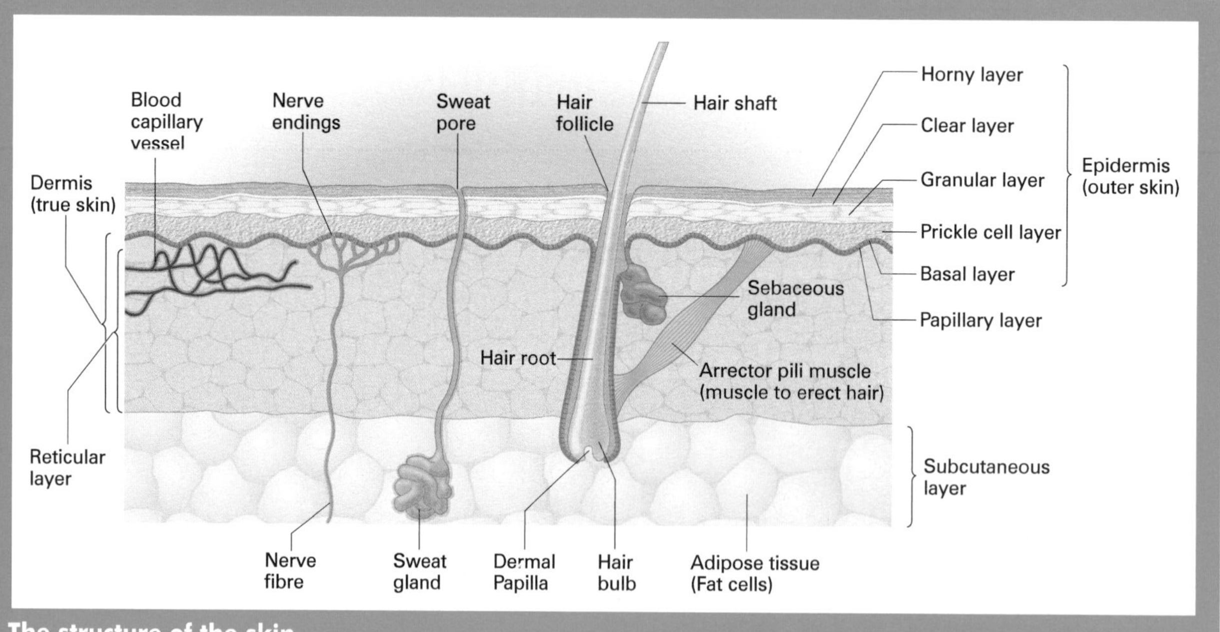

The structure of the skin

The skin's functions

Sense and feeling

The nerve endings in our skin are very sensitive. They pick up changes in temperature or pressure, and alert us to pain.

Heat control

Skin helps to control the temperature in the body – how hot or cold we are.

- When we are hot, we begin to sweat through sweat glands in the skin, and this cools us down.
- When we are cold, the muscles that are joined to the hairs in our skin tighten up causing goose pimples and we begin to shiver, which warms up our body.

Protection

Skin is like a waterproof jacket – it protects the body from the weather, dirt, bacteria and injury. To keep the outer layers smooth and soft and free of splits and cracks that would let germs enter, the skin produces water from the pores and oil from the oil glands.

Vitamin-making

When we are outside, the sun's rays on the skin produce vitamin D for the body. This vitamin is needed for strong bones and teeth.

Storage

The skin stores fat and water, without which we could not survive.

Waste removal

Some waste products and toxins are removed from the body through our sweat.

toxins: poisons

Why we apply make-up

We apply make-up to alter or improve a person's appearance by using colour, shape and shading.

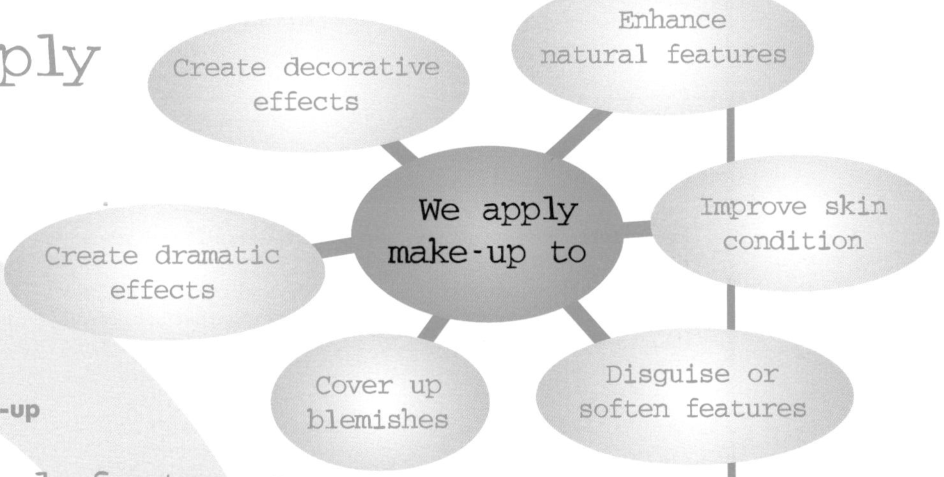

We apply make-up to
- Enhance natural features
- Improve skin condition
- Disguise or soften features
- Cover up blemishes
- Create dramatic effects
- Create decorative effects

Reasons for applying make-up

Enhance natural features

Every face has its good points. We can enhance our natural features, such as long eyelashes and high cheekbones, with make-up techniques. When you look at pictures of fashion models they look beautiful, but without the skills of a make-up artist and the use of make-up products, they would look very different.

enhance: make more attractive

TRY IT OUT!

Write down other ways that would help you to improve a client's natural features.

TOPTIP

Make the most of our good features: **Eye lashes** use an eyelash curler and mascara with build-up fibres. **Eye colour** use a contrasting colour to the eyes. **Lips** apply lip liner to even out the shape

contrasting: different

Disguise or soften features or cover up blemishes

Few of us have a perfect face shape. The most desirable shape is usually oval. Make-up can be used to alter parts of our appearance – this is called corrective make-up. With the use of darker foundation, clever highlighters and blusher, it is possible to create the illusion of a different face shape.

appearance

Corrective make-up:

- Reduces bad points.
- Improves good points.
- Uses light colours to highlight or show up features.
- Uses dark colours to conceal features.

hide

Corrective make-up for different face shapes

The pictures below will guide you on how best to shade or highlight each type of face shape.

Shader

Highlighter

Blusher

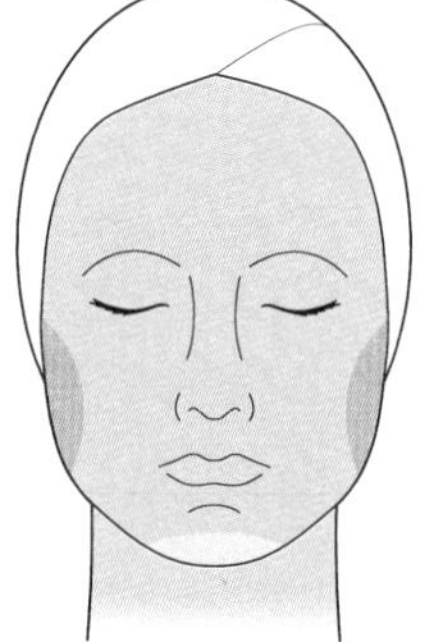

Round face: Shade under the cheekbones. Highlight the chin to make the face seem longer. Use blusher just under the cheekbones.

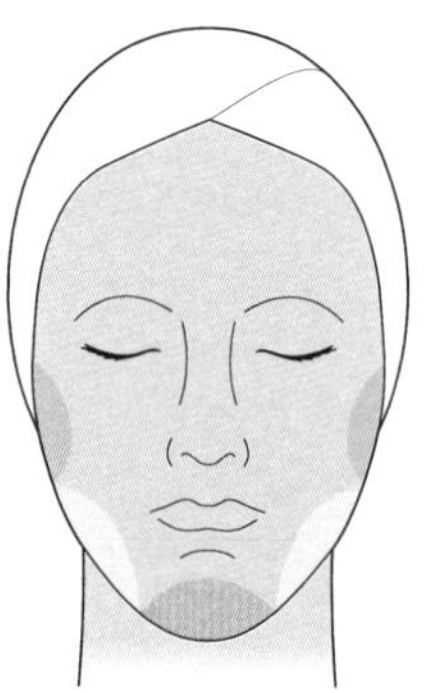

Heart-shaped face: Shade the chin. Highlight the sides of the chin to balance out the shape and make the chin look wider. Use blusher on the cheekbones.

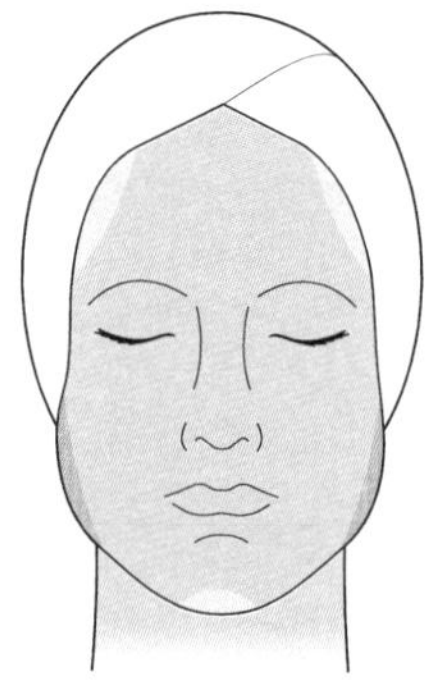

Triangular face: Highlight the sides of the forehead to show it up more. Shade the jaw area to make it look smaller. Use blusher on the cheekbones.

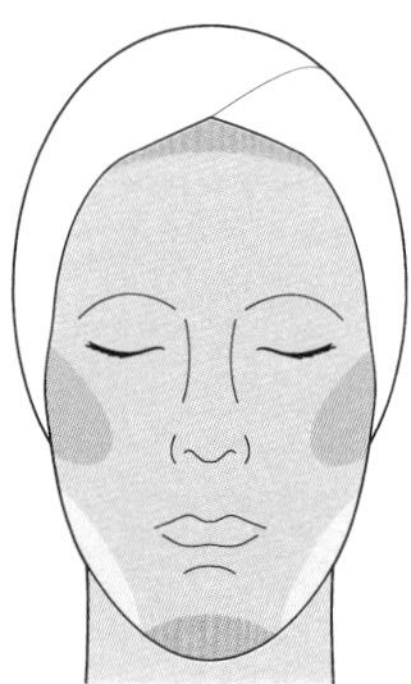

Oblong face: Shade the forehead and chin. Perhaps highlight the cheekbones. Use blusher just at the sides of the cheekbone, near the temples.

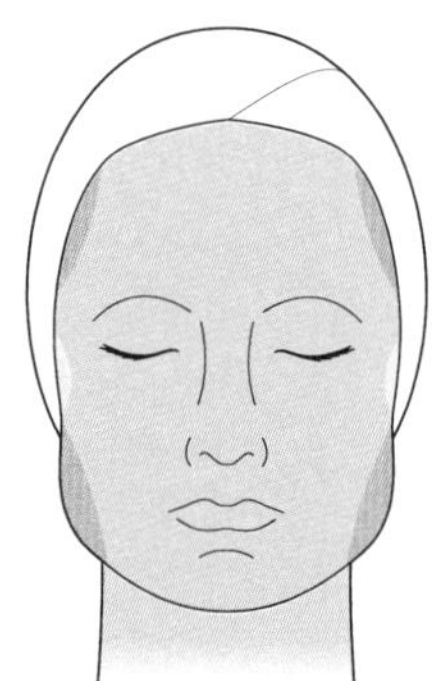

Square face: Shade all the corners to soften the angles. Highlight the outer part of the cheekbones.

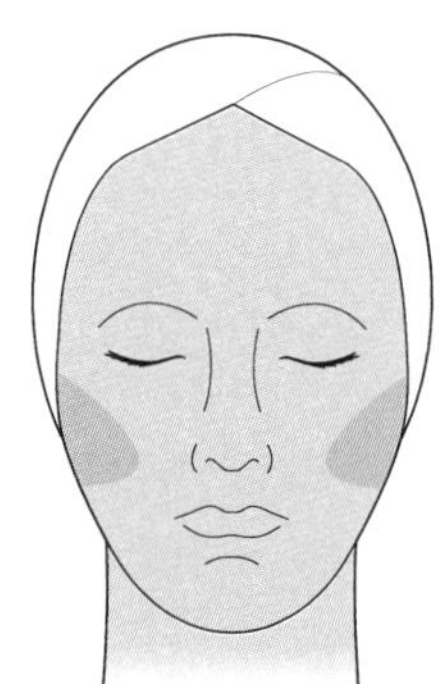

Oval face: The 'perfect' face shape – requires no correction!

Corrective make-up for the eyes

Dark colours tend to make the eyes appear smaller whereas bright colours emphasise them.

show up

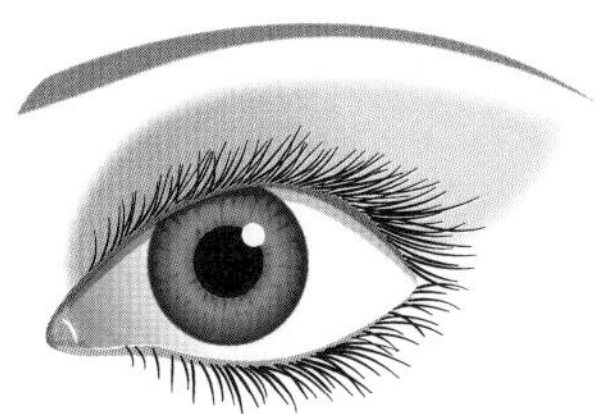

Wide-apart eyes: Apply darker shades on the inside and lighter shades on the outside.

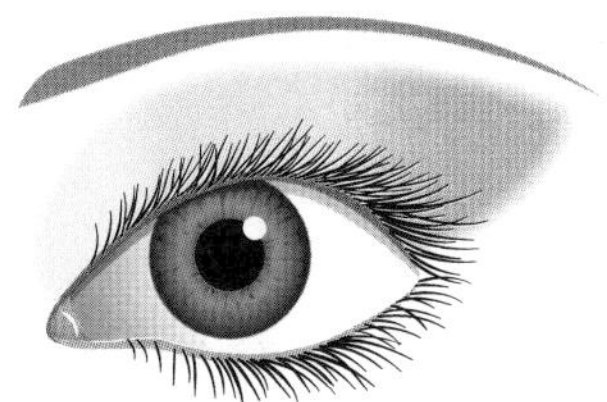

Close set eyes: Apply lighter colour on the inner eye and darker shades on the outer eye.

TRY IT OUT!

Discuss with your tutor how you could correct small eyes and deep-set eyes. Draw pictures to show how you would do this.

TOPTIP

Take care to apply the lip liner quite finely. If it is too heavily applied, it can make the lips look worse than before you started!

Corrective make-up for the lips

Cover the lips with foundation. Using lip liner, draw in the outline of the shape that you would like the lips to have, then fill in the shape with lipstick.

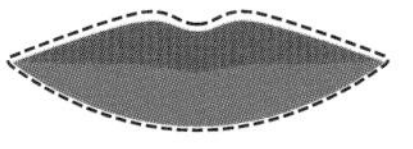

Thin lips: Apply lip liner just outside of the natural lip line and add a lighter colour of lipstick in the centre of the lips. This will give the lips the appearance of being full.

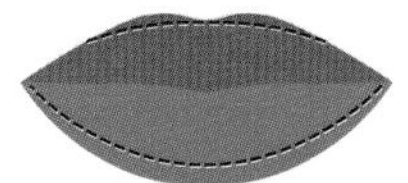

Full lips: Apply lip liner just inside the natural lip line to make the lips look thinner.

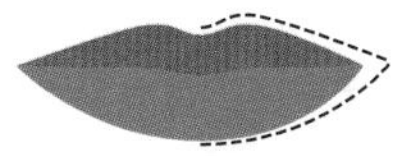

Uneven lips: Correct the uneven parts – where it is thinner or thicker – by drawing around the lip with lip liner.

Corrective make-up for noses

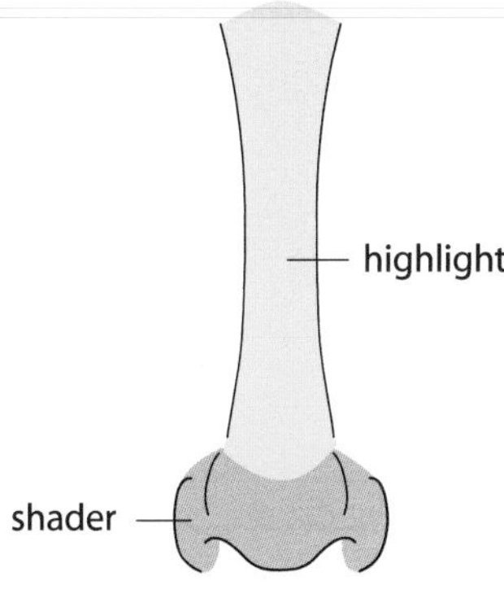

Long nose: Shade the tip to shorten.

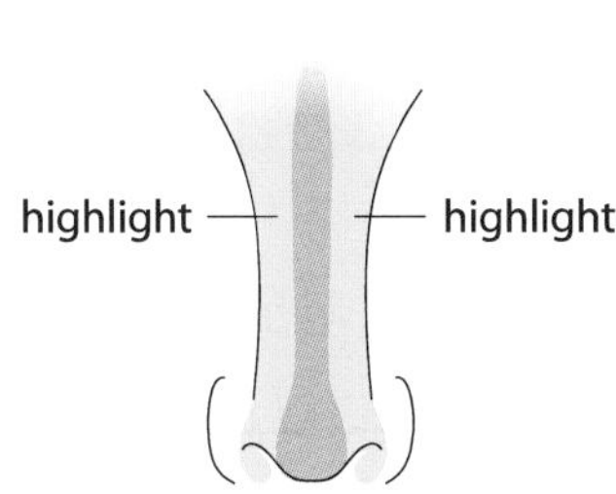

Short, thin nose: Highlight the sides to make the nose appear wider, which will in turn make it appear less short.

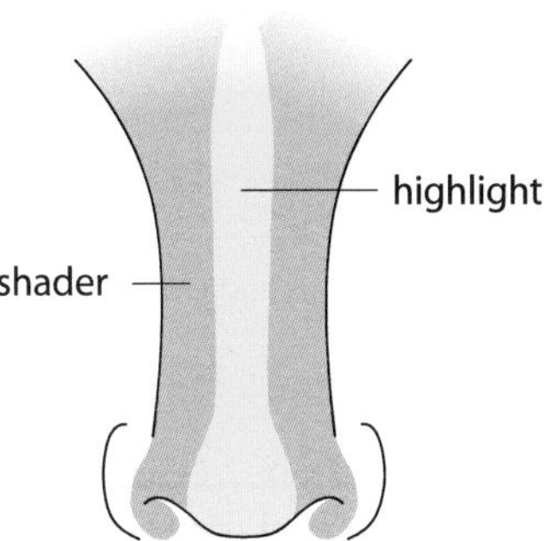

Wide nose: Shade the sides.

Create dramatic and decorative effects

The make-up used on the catwalk, in the theatre, on TV or film and in glossy magazines is usually heavily applied and long lasting. It is used to create special effects ranging from high fashion to fantasy or theatrical looks. It is expertly applied and very artistic, which can give gloss and glamour or even alter the appearance of a performer for the stage or screen.

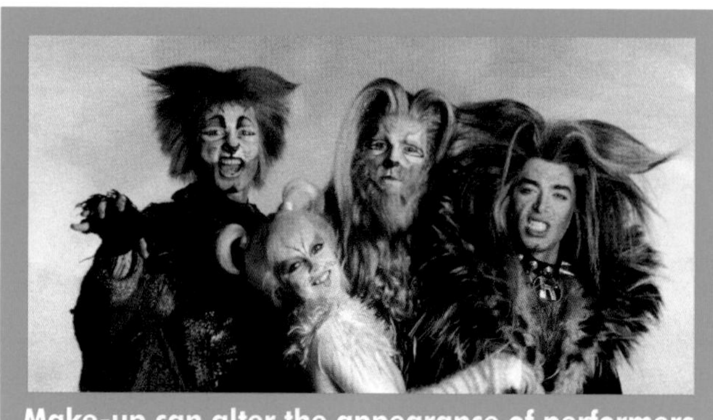

Make-up can alter the appearance of performers

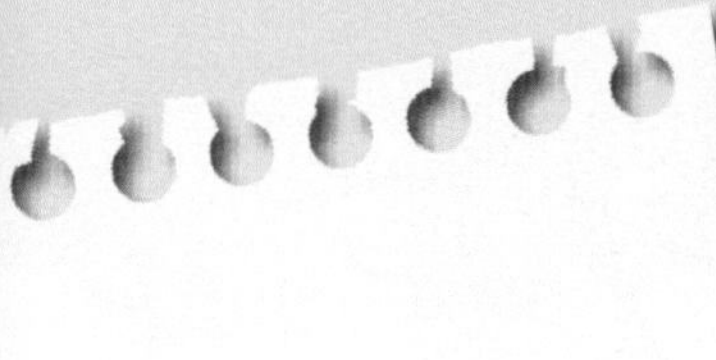

OVER TO YOU...

Find pictures of make-up products, designs and techniques that could be used for fantasy make-up. They could be from magazines, advertisements, sketches or photographs of make-up treatments that you have carried out. Add them to your portfolio or scrapbook.

Day make-up

A natural looking, day make-up can be one of the most difficult to do as it needs to look as though the person is wearing hardly any make-up after you have applied it. At the same time, if you were to look at photos of before and after, you must be able to see an improvement. Each step of the make-up routine is applied lightly and should be very well blended.

Evening make-up

This is more adventurous than day make-up. Deeper, brighter colours are used, as gentle colours look washed out in bright lights. Extra cosmetics you could use, depending on the occasion, are:

- False eyelashes.
- Glitter.
- Lip gloss.
- Sparkle powders.
- Glitter body and hair sprays.

Improve skin condition

Make-up can help the skin in various ways:

- It can protect the skin against the effects of weather and pollution.
- Foundation evens out the texture and colour of the natural skin, especially if it is blotchy and uneven.
- Lipsticks keep lips soft and supple, especially lipsticks with added moisturisers.

Skin types, conditions, disorders and reactions

Client consultation

Before starting the treatment, you should carry out a client consultation, which will involve analysing the client's face shape and skin.

First, lay the client in a semi-reclined position, then stand in front of her to decide what face shape she has (look back at page 136 to remind you of the various face shapes).

semi-reclined: lying back but not completely flat

Next, you will need to cleanse the client's face before carrying out the skin analysis. A skin analysis should only be done on clean skin and involves checking the client's:

- Skin type.
- Skin condition and problem areas.
- Allergies.

Write everything you find out on the client's record card, which should include the following information:

- The treatment that the client would like.
- The results of the skin analysis.
- Any allergies.
- Any contra-indications (see When not to carry out a make-up on page 140).
- The type of make-up she wants.

contra-indications: reasons why you cannot treat the client

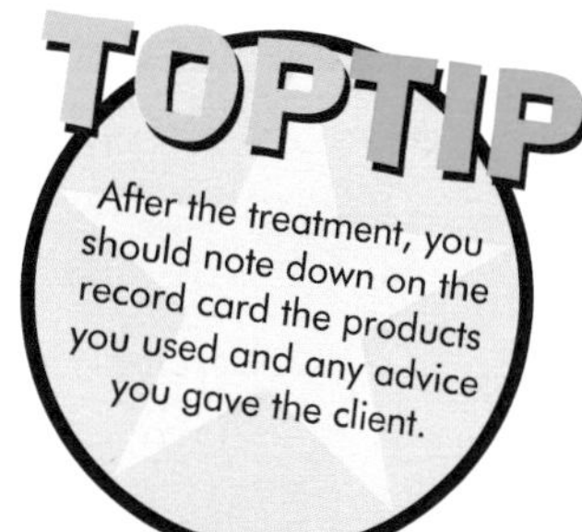

TOPTIP
After the treatment, you should note down on the record card the products you used and any advice you gave the client.

Skin types

Normal skin

Normal skin is a rare skin type, usually found in children and young people.

Normal skin:

- Is smooth and clear with no blemishes.
- Feels soft to the touch.
- Has very tiny pores that are difficult to see.

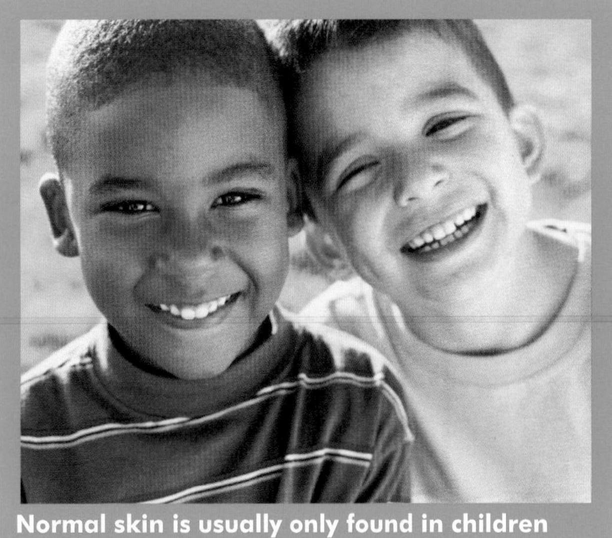

Normal skin is usually only found in children

Oily skin

Oily skin is caused when the skin produces too much oil. Although we need oil to keep our skin smooth, if the skin produces too much oil, this can cause problems. Oily skin:

- Has a shiny complexion with blackheads and blemishes.
- Has quite large pores.
- Can be quite thick.

This type of skin can start or worsen in teenagers when puberty hormones are at their most active.

puberty hormones: chemicals in the body that cause bodily changes

Dry skin

Dry skin lacks oil because the oil glands in the skin do not produce enough. Dry skin:

- Feels tight.
- May flake and chap easily after washing, especially if soap is used.
- Soaks up creams and lotions easily.
- Can become lined and wrinkled early (especially around the eyes).

This type of skin must be moisturised well.

softened by the use of creams

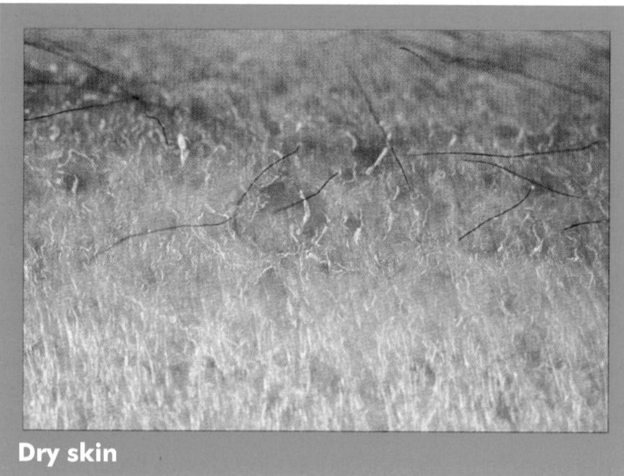

Dry skin

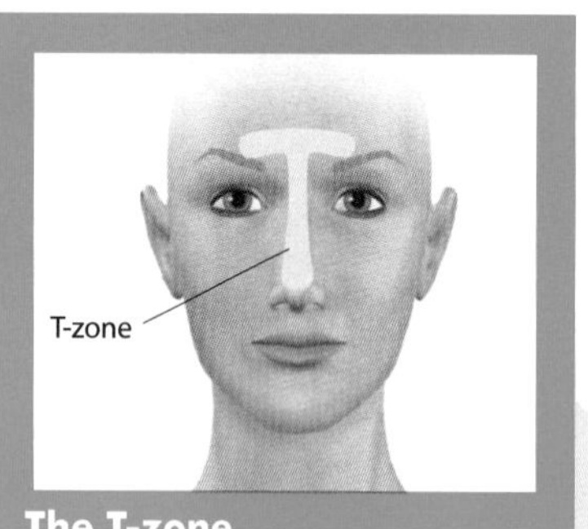

The T-zone

Combination skin

Combination skin is made up of two skin types. These types vary, but the most common is normal or dry skin on the cheek area and an oily part on the nose and across the forehead (known as the T-zone). The oily T-zone shows up as a shiny nose and forehead with blackheads.

When not to carry out a make-up

Contra-indications

Whenever you treat a client you will need to be aware of conditions that might prevent you carrying out the make-up. Conditions that cannot be treated are called contra-indications. It could be unsafe to treat a client with a contra-indication.

Contra-indications include:

- Blisters around the mouth and nose, e.g. a cold sore.
- Bloodshot and watery eyes, e.g. an eye infection.
- Redness – this could be a sign of an allergy, sunburn or an injury.
- Swelling or lumps – this could be bruising or something more serious.
- Dry, red and flaky skin, which could be eczema or dermatitis (sore, very dry skin conditions).
- Healing scars.
- Cuts.

If you notice anything unusual on the skin, you should ask your tutor to check before you start the treatment as some conditions may be infectious.

able to pass from person to person

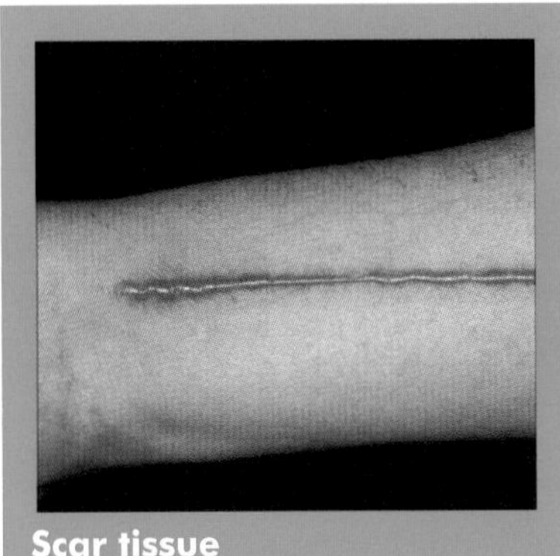
Scar tissue

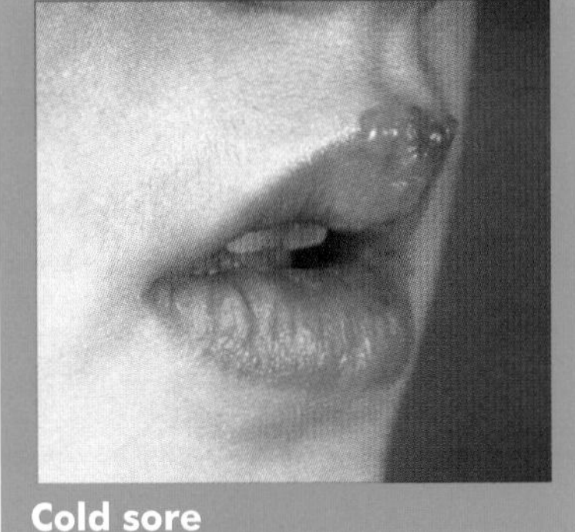
Cold sore

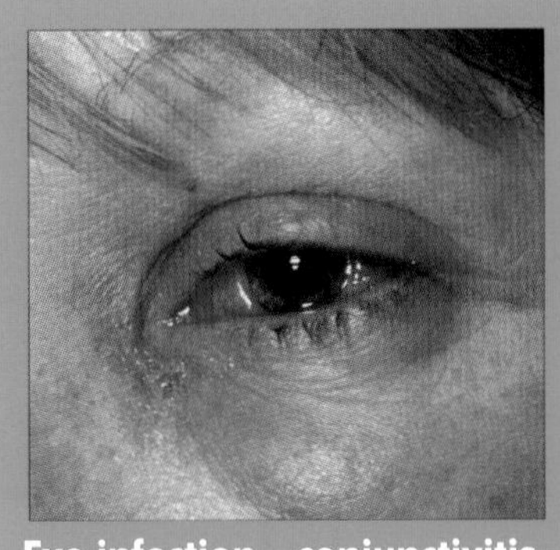
Eye infection – conjunctivitis

Some contra-indications

salon scene

Femi had just started her work experience at a local beauty salon. On her first day, she watched the therapist Jo carry out a make-up treatment. Femi, Jo and the client went to the treatment room. Jo cleansed, toned and moisturised the client's skin but, as the make-up came off, Femi thought she could see a sore at the corner of the client's mouth. Femi thought the sore looked like a cold sore and asked Jo about it. Jo said it would be all right as the make-up would cover it up.

While Jo was completing the make-up, Femi also noticed that the brushes were dirty, the lipstick was used straight onto the lips and Jo used her fingers to blend eye shadow. Powdered make-up also fell onto the client's jumper.

What did Jo do wrong?

What could happen if you treat a client with a contra-indication?

Do you think that the client will be pleased with her treatment? Explain your answer.

What did Femi learn from watching the treatment?

Allergies

Another reason why you might not be able to carry out a make-up is if the client has an allergy to a cosmetic product. Some cosmetics contain ingredients that could cause an allergic skin reaction, as shown in the table on page 142.

sensitivity

Ingredients in cosmetic products that could cause an allergic reaction

Products	Ingredients that could cause a reaction
Skin care	Soaps and perfumes
Creams and lotions	Lanolin (a natural oil that comes from sheep's wool) generally used in cheaper creams and lotions
Lipsticks, face powders and blushers	Dyes and colourings
Eye shadows	Powdered crushed glass (used to add shimmer)
Mascara and eyeliner	Alcohol and fibres
Toning lotions	Alcohol or citrus ingredients
Nail polish and removers	Acetone and alcohol

To check if a client has any known allergies, ask her:

- Have you ever had an allergic reaction to cosmetics, nail varnishes or skin care products?
- Do you suffer from hayfever, eczema or dermatitis?
- Is your skin sensitive to touch, heat or cold?

If the client answers 'yes' to any of the above questions, it means she has a sensitive skin that could react badly to some products. You will then need to seek further advice from your tutor.

Always check for allergies before applying make-up. Some clients may be allergic to plants and flowers or may have food allergies, which may mean they are sensitive to other things too.

Even though you check for allergies before the treatment, some clients may still react badly to a product by showing one or several of the following signs:

- Itching.
- Tightness.
- Blistering.
- Watery eyes.
- Excess perspiration.
- Swelling.
- Redness.

All cosmetics must have their ingredients listed on them. Make sure you check them if your client has a known allergy.

If this happens, remove the product immediately, bathe the skin with clean, cool water and advise the client to seek medical advice before using the product again.

sweating

Products, materials and equipment for make-up treatments

Before starting a treatment, you will need to be well prepared. All products, materials and equipment should be to hand and your work area and equipment should be clean and tidy.

Products to prepare the skin for a make-up treatment

Product	Type	Uses
Eye make-up remover	Oil, lotion or gel. Use an oil-based remover on waterproof mascara and heavy make-up.	Mild cleaning product that dissolves eye make-up without rubbing the eyes.
Cleanser	**Cream** – thick cleanser for dry or mature skin types. Dissolves make-up quickly. **Milk** – thin, runny cleanser for most skin types, except very dry skin. Ideal for young or normal skin types, but not very good at removing heavy or waterproof make-up. **Lotion** – similar in thickness to a milk cleanser. Contains antibacterial ingredients to help spotty and combination skins.	Removes make-up. Cleans dirt and dust grime from the skin and pores. Removes oil and dead skin cells.
Toner	Available in different strengths and chosen depending on the skin type. Use stronger toners, known as astringents, to dry out oily, problem skins.	Removes any left-over cleanser from the skin. Dissolves oil. Refreshes and cools the skin. Tightens the skin and pores.
Moisturiser	**Cream** – for dry skins **Lotion** – for oily skins **Milk** – for young, normal or sensitive skins.	Softens and protects the skin's surface. Rehydrates the skin. Provides a smooth base for applying make-up.

antibacterial: reduces the spread of germs

rehydrates: adds water or moisture.

A good set of brushes is essential for a professional make-up. Each stage of the make-up needs a different brush.

Brushes

Type	Uses
Face powder brush	The largest brush, used to apply or blend face powder.
Blusher brush	Used to apply blusher onto the cheek area.
Contour brush	Used for shading and highlighting the cheeks and face when doing corrective make-up.
Eyebrow brush	Consists of a brush on one side for brushing brows into shape and a comb on the other side for separating lashes.
Sponge applicator	Used for applying colour to the eye lids.
Eye shadow brush	Used for shading and blending eye shadow.
Angled eye shadow brush	Used to apply colour or blend colour on the edges or sockets of the eyes.
Fluff brush	Completes the blending as it is very soft and will remove any unblended edges.
Eyeliner brush	Used to apply eyeliner or for blending eye pencil.
Lip liner brush	Used to apply lipstick smoothly.

Materials for a make-up treatment

Materials	Uses
Cotton buds	Used to correct mistakes or make-up smudges.
Eye pads (cotton wool circles or squares)	Placed on the eye while using a magnifying lamp for skin analysis.
Damp cotton wool half moons	Placed under the bottom lashes to protect the skin under the eyes while make-up is cleansed off.
Damp cotton wool squares	Used to cleanse the face.
Tissues	Used to blot excess toner, moisturiser and the first coat of lipstick.
Dry cotton wool	Used to cover the tip of the orange stick.
Couch roll	Used to protect the client's clothing.
Sponge wedges	Used to apply foundation to the skin.
Make-up cape	Protects the client's upper clothes from make-up spills.
Headband or turban	Used to protect the client's hair from products and to prevent hair getting in the way of the treatment.
Bowls	For holding cotton wool, tissue and the client's jewellery.
Waste bin	A pedal bin with a lid is best for hygiene purposes.
Spatula	A wide wooden stick that is used to scoop out cream or lotions from pots.
Orange sticks	Used to remove make-up. Cotton wool is wrapped around the ends to soften the tips for safety when cleaning around the eyes.
Palette	Used for decanting products and for mixing colours.
Sharpener	Used to sharpen lip and eye pencils.

decanting: pouring from one container to another

Make-up products

Product	Uses
Concealer	Covers blemishes or shadows under the eyes.
Foundation	Smoothes out the colour of the skin and provides a base for the rest of the make-up.
Powder	Sets the foundation and prevents shine.
Blusher	Adds soft colour to the cheeks and shape to the face.
Eye shadow	Gives glamour and colour to the eyes, also good for shaping and correcting eyes.
Eyeliner	Opens, lengthens or emphasises the eyes.
Eyebrow pencil	Defines the eyebrow's natural shape, darkens the brow or fills in where the brow is thin.
Mascara	Makes the lashes look fuller and longer.
Lip liner	Evens out the shape of the lips and helps lipstick stay on longer.
Lipstick	Adds colour to the lips.
Lip gloss	Adds gloss and shine to the lips. It can be used on top of lipstick or on its own.
Face paints	Used to create fantasy make-up.

marks out

Preparing the skin

1. Cleanse eyes. Place a cotton wool half moon under the eye to stop the make-up staining the skin. Apply eye make-up remover to the lid using gentle circular movements. Stroke downwards with a clean, damp piece of cotton wool to remove the make-up. Repeat until all the eye make-up is removed.

2. Cleanse lips. Apply cleanser to the lips in small circles, using your little finger. Support one side of the mouth and sweep across with a clean piece of cotton wool from one side to the other and back again.

3. First facial cleanse. Follow the cleansing routine (see below). Remove cleanser with damp cotton wool squares.

4. Skin analysis. Look carefully at the skin to find out the skin type, condition and texture.

5. Second facial cleanse. Follow the cleansing routine (see below). Remove cleanser with damp cotton wool squares.

6. Apply toner. Put onto damp cotton wool and follow the cleansing

7. Blot toner. Using a split tissue, place it on the skin to soak up the excess toner.

8. Repeat toning and blotting.

9. Apply moisturiser. Use cleansing routine strokes.

Preparing the skin for a make-up treatment

Now leave the skin to settle for five minutes and to give the moisturiser time to sink in.

Cleansing routine

Decant enough cleanser onto your hand to complete the cleanse. Spread the cleanser between both hands and start the cleansing routine:

1. 4 stroking effleurage on the neck

2. 4 stroking effleurage on the right cheek

3. 4 stroking effleurage on the chin

4. 4 stroking effleurage on the left cheek

5. Circles around the chin

6. Move upwards keeping in contact with the skin – do not lift your hands off

7. Petrissage circles around the mouth and nose

8. 4 stroking effleurage on the bridge of the nose

9. 4 stroking effleurage on the forehead

10. 4 eye circles (go in the direction of the eyebrow)

11. Finish with pressure on the temples before lifting off hands

The cleansing routine

effleurage means 'to flow', so these are stroking, smooth massage movements

petrissage means 'to knead', so these are circling, kneading massage movements

TRY IT OUT!

Find out about other massage movements that are used.

Applying make-up products

TOPTIP
A little foundation goes a long way!

Foundation

Choosing the correct foundation is essential. The foundation should provide a smooth, even base to work on and should be as close to the natural skin tone as possible. You should test the colour on the jaw line. Two colours can be blended together to get the correct colour if necessary. There are many types of foundation and the type you use will depend on the skin type of the client.

Application: Decant some foundation onto your palette. Use the make-up sponge wedge to apply it to the face using downward and outward strokes. This avoids disturbing the tiny hairs on the face, which could make the foundation go blotchy. Blend the foundation well and fade it out at the jaw line to prevent hard lines.

Dear Nat

When I apply foundation I can never get it exactly the same colour as the skin. It looks as if the client has a line along her chin, and her neck looks a different colour to her face. I have six foundation colours to choose from.

From Maria

Nat says

Believe it or not, there are many different skin tones, and every one is different! Try decanting a small amount of each foundation colour onto your palette. Use a clean orange stick to mix together two different colours to try to get a closer match to the skin tone.

Concealer

Concealer can be applied before or after foundation depending on the type and how many blemishes, scars or shadows need to be covered up. Concealer is available in sticks, tubes or jars and can also be medicated for use with spots. Concealer is thicker than foundation.

medicated: containing a healing ingredient

Application: Scrape a small amount of concealer onto a spatula. Apply to the skin using a brush, dotting in the required place. Then using clean fingertips, blend gradually.

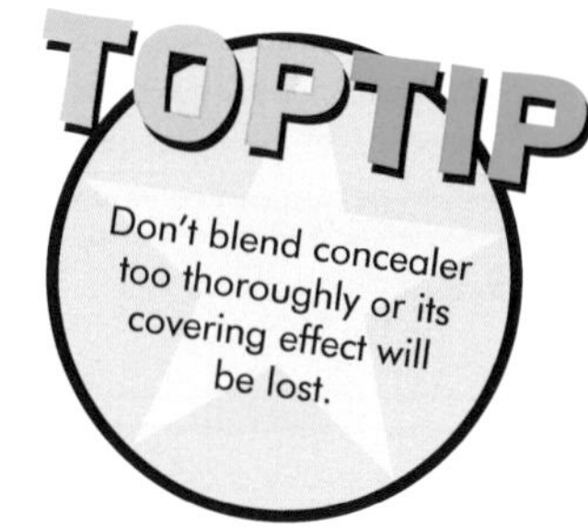

TOPTIP
Don't blend concealer too thoroughly or its covering effect will be lost.

Powder

This is used to set the foundation, make it last longer and to cut down shine. Powder comes in loose form or in a compact. Some powders contain glitter or pearlised ingredients, which are great for evening make-up. Use a good match to the foundation or use a translucent or transparent one which is suitable for all.

Application: Apply loose powder with cotton wool using a pressing rolling action over the foundation. A large soft brush then needs to be used to brush off extra powder from the face so that it does not look thick.

Eye shadow

This comes in many forms in a wide range of colours and textures. Eye shadow brings colour to the face and can lessen the effect of less attractive facial features. Eye make-up can be used to correct faults such as deep-set eyes. Effects can be soft or dramatic depending on the client's wishes or occasion. It is not necessary to use the same colour as the eyes as they naturally contain many different flecks of colour. Avoid shiny colours on wrinkled skin.

Application: Apply with a sponge applicator or soft brush. The lightest shade, the highlighter is applied under the brow and the darker shadow colours on the lid. Eye shadow must be blended well to give a soft appearance and professional finish.

Work with care around the eyes as they are very delicate

Eyeliner

Eyeliner is used to draw attention to the eyes. It can be used to open, lengthen or add depth to the eyes depending on the type of application and colour. There are many types – liquid, cake and pencil or pen applicator.

Application: Apply in a fine line as close to the roots of the lashes as possible. It can be applied either to the top or bottom lashes or both. To prevent hard lines, blend into eye shadow by applying eye shadow softly over the top. Use a damp, cotton wool bud to clean up any smudges or mistakes.

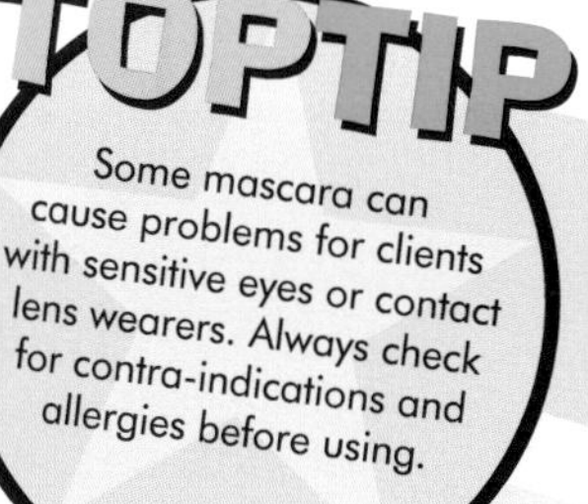

TOPTIP
Some mascara can cause problems for clients with sensitive eyes or contact lens wearers. Always check for contra-indications and allergies before using.

Mascara

Mascara makes the lashes look fuller and longer and comes in many colours and types, for example some have fibres or are waterproof.

Application: Apply downwards over the upper lashes first, then ask client to look up slightly and stroke the lashes upwards to coat underneath. Then coat the lower lashes. Keep a clean mascara comb so that you can separate any lashes that join together. Apply mascara in several thin coats rather than one thick coat, and allow to dry between coats.

Blusher

This gives soft colour to the cheeks, creates better shape and can correct face shape.

Application: Apply powder blusher after the powder, cream blushers before powder. Apply with a brush to the cheek area, building up the colour slowly until you are happy with the result. Heavily applied blusher looks unnatural.

Lip liner

This is used to give a smooth outline to the lips and to correct their shape. Use a colour close to the natural lip colour if using a pale lipstick or clear lip gloss. If using a brighter lipstick, use a lip liner of the same colour as the lipstick.

Application: Rest your little finger on the client's chin for support and gently outline the lips with the pencil. Do not ask the client to stretch her lips because when they relax and go back to normal the liner will be uneven and too dark.

Lipstick

This is the final touch to a make-up and brings the whole effect together. It adds colour and texture to the face as well as gloss and shine to the lips. Lipstick comes in many colours and textures, ranging from cream to pearlised and matt to glossy.

Application: Scrape a little off the stick with a spatula and apply using a lip brush. Coat the outer part of the lips first and then fill in the centre. Blot with a tissue and then apply a second coat – this will give a better coverage and will make the lipstick last longer.

Lip gloss

If applied to bare lips, lip gloss gives a beautiful sheen, or if used on top of lipstick, it enhances the lipstick. It comes in many forms and colours.

Application: Apply evenly with a lip brush, taking care not to overload the lips.

Face paints

These are water-based paints that come in many colours and are easily applied and removed. They are used to paint animal, insect or character designs onto faces and sometimes the body.

Application: Apply using a damp sponge for the base colour. Keep fresh clean water nearby to rinse colour from the sponge before using a different colour. When lines or drawings are needed, a brush can be used over the base colour.

TRY IT OUT!

Find pictures of make-up on celebrities in magazines. Label the ones you like and say why. Do the same for the ones that you do not like.

Always work with clean, sterilised equipment to prevent germs spreading. Don't blow on your make-up brushes as you will be blowing germs onto them.

How to apply day make-up

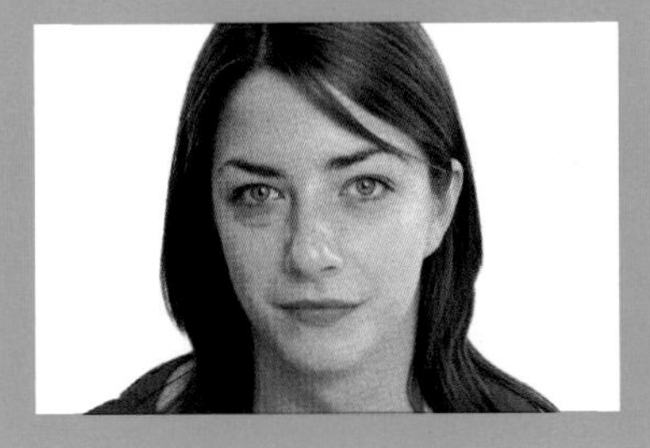

1 Before day make-up is applied.

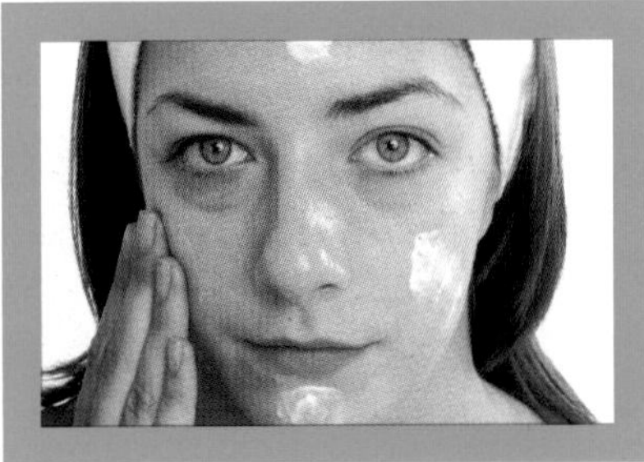

2 Remove make-up and cleanse and moisturise face.

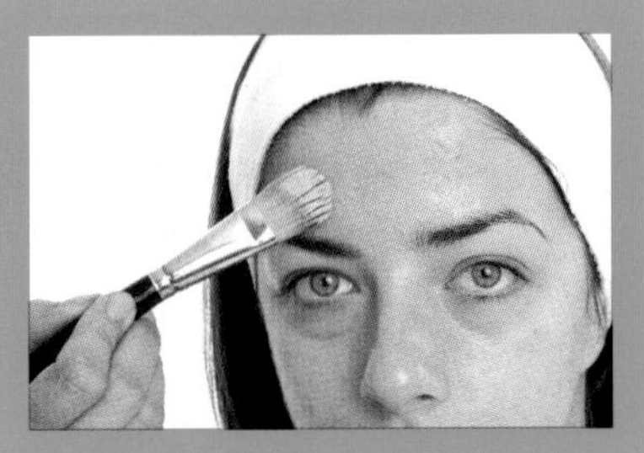

3 Apply foundation with a brush or a sponge wedge moving downwards and outwards.

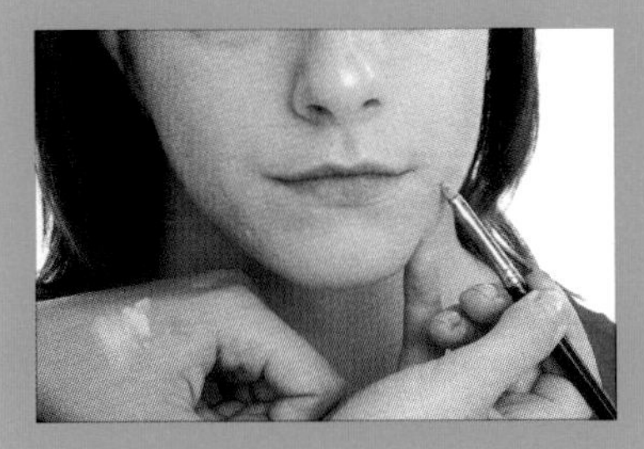

4 Apply concealer with a small brush and use a clean finger to blend it in.

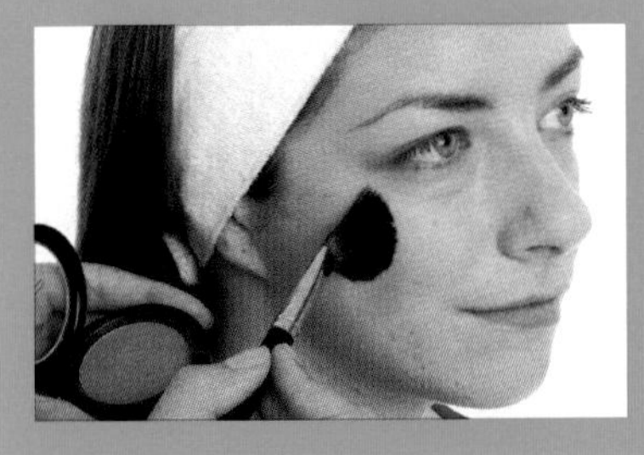

5 Apply powder with a powder brush to set the foundation. Apply blusher with a blusher brush.

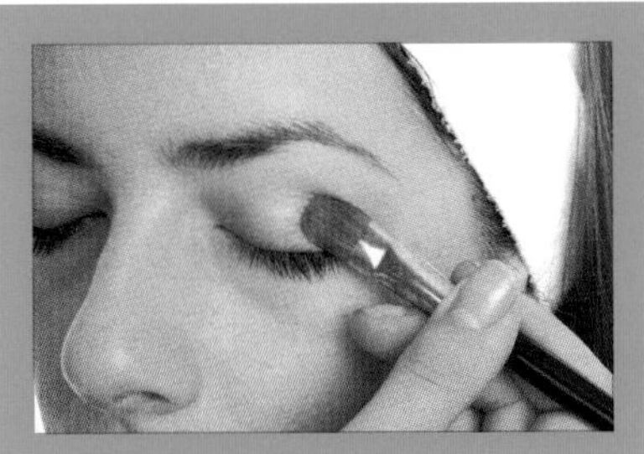

6 Apply eye shadow using an eye shadow brush. Apply mascara.

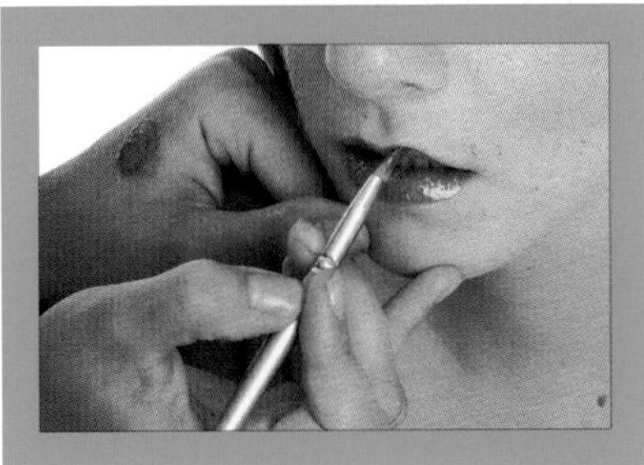

7 Complete the look by applying lipstick and lip gloss with a lip liner brush.

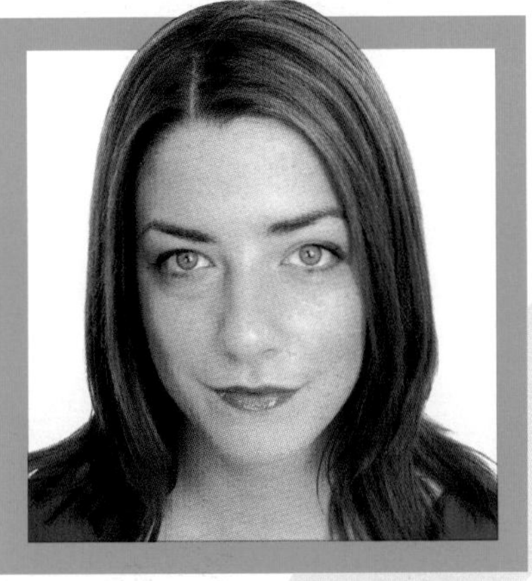

8 The finished result!

OVER TO YOU...

Find pictures of make-up products, designs and techniques that could be used for day make-up. They could be from magazines, advertisements, sketches or photographs of make-up treatments that you have carried out. Add them to your portfolio or scrapbook.

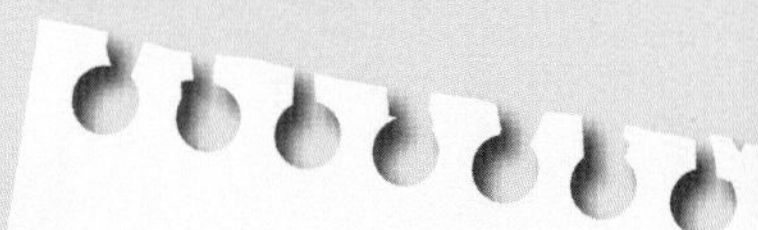

How to apply evening make-up

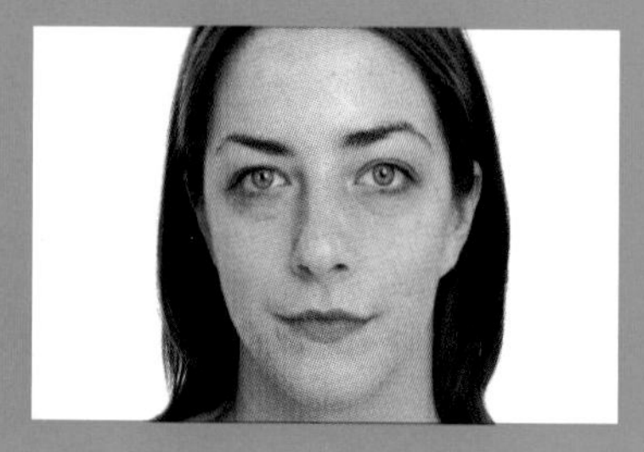

1 Before evening make-up is applied.

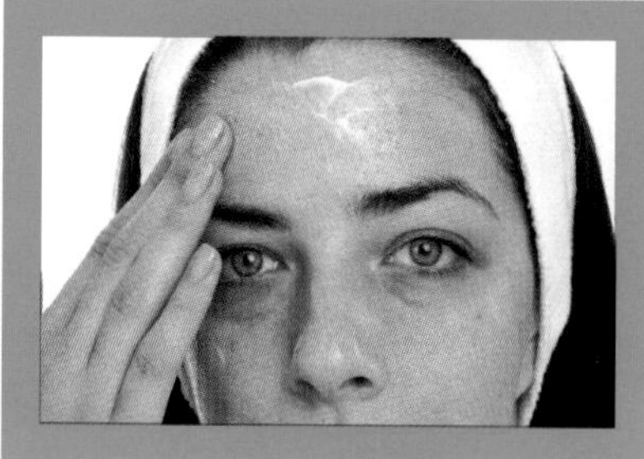

2 Remove make-up and cleanse and moisturise face.

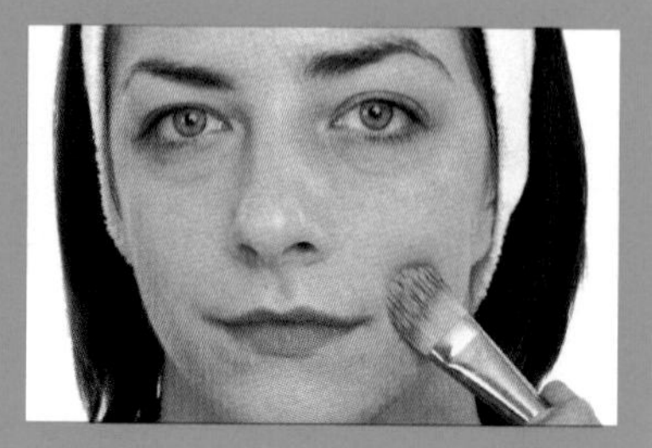

3 Apply foundation with a brush or sponge wedge moving downwards and outwards.

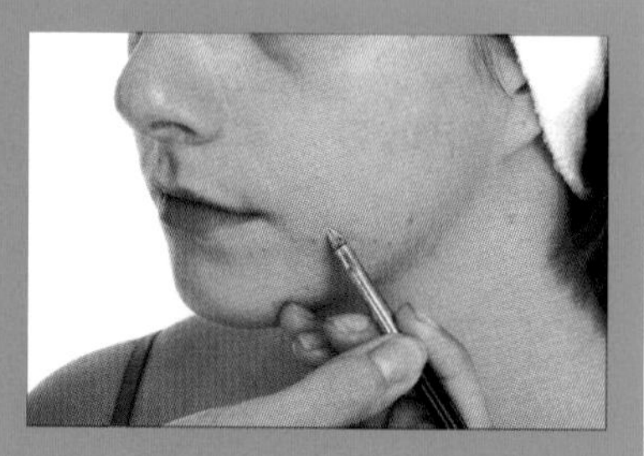

4 Apply concealer with a small brush and use a clean finger to blend it in.

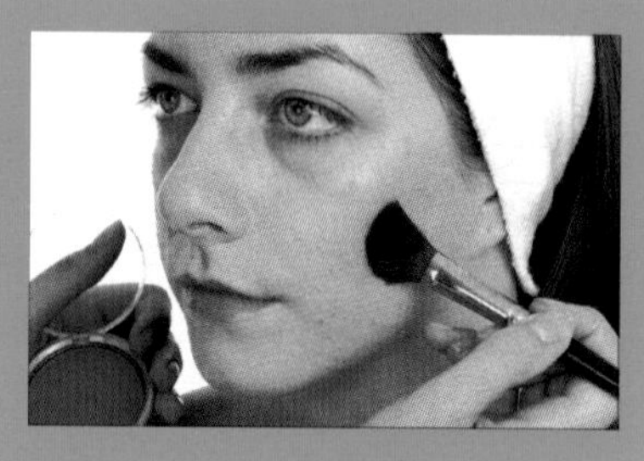

5 Apply blusher and shimmer with a blusher brush. Apply powder.

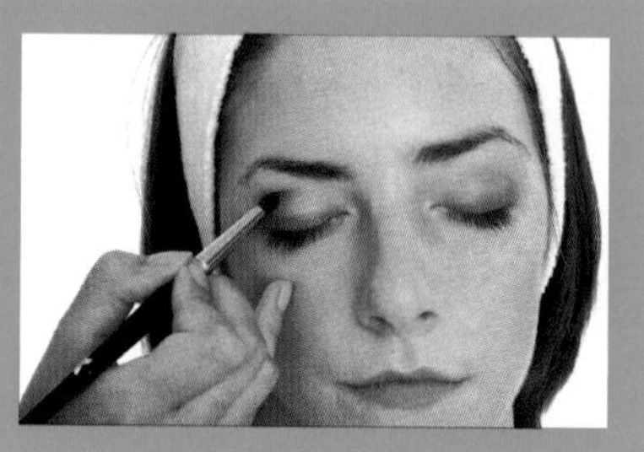

6 Apply eye shadow using an eye shadow brush. Then apply mascara to the lashes using even, light strokes and comb through with the comb side of the eyebrow brush to separate the lashes.

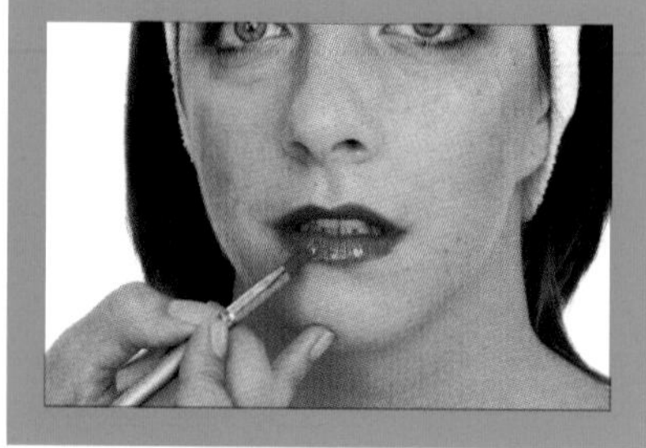

7 Complete the look by applying lipstick and lip gloss with a lip liner brush.

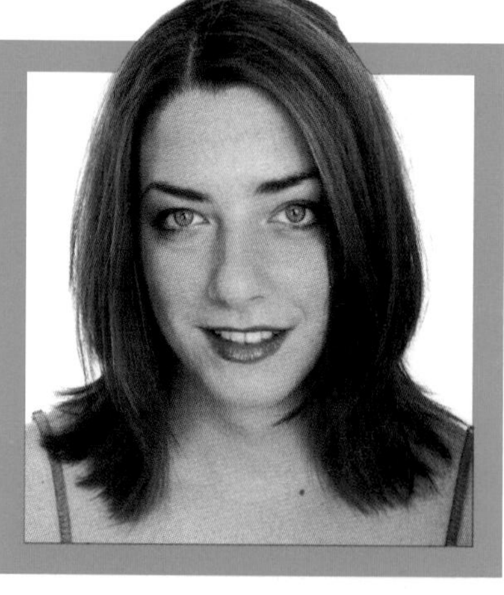

8 The finished result!

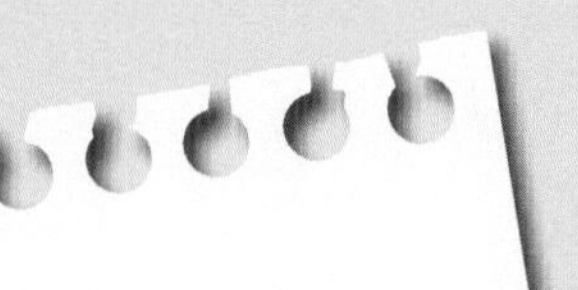

OVER TO YOU...

Find pictures of make-up products, designs and techniques that could be used for evening make-up. They could be from magazines, advertisements, sketches or photographs of make-up treatments that you have carried out. Add them to your portfolio or scrapbook.

OVER TO YOU...

Find pictures of make-up products, designs and techniques that could be used for bridal make-up. They could be from magazines, advertisements, sketches or photographs of make-up treatments that you have carried out. Add them to your portfolio or scrapbook.

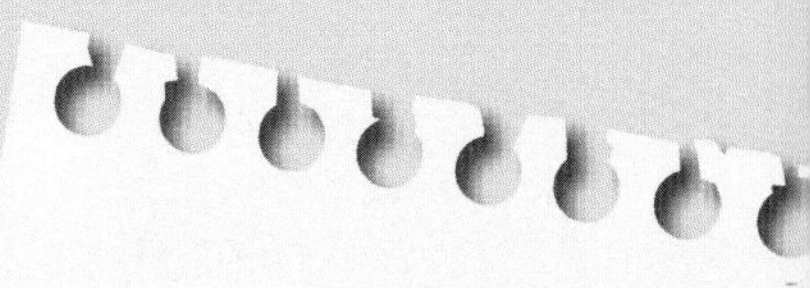

Check what you know...

1. The skin has how many main layers?

☐ 1 ☐ 2 ☐ 3

2. The skin stores:

☐ the sun's rays
☐ vitamin C
☐ fat and water

3. What is the main purpose of applying make-up?

☐ to match the colour of the client's clothes
☐ to alter or improve a person's appearance by using colour, shape and shading
☐ to make the skin waterproof

4. What are the three stages to a clean skin?

☐ tone, moisturise and blot
☐ moisturise, cleanse and tone
☐ cleanse, tone and moisturise

5. Your client's skin unexpectedly reacts to a make-up product. What should you do?

☐ call a first aider
☐ remove the product immediately and bathe the skin with clean, cool water
☐ carry on with the treatment

6. What is the purpose of a headband or turban during a make-up treatment?

☐ to keep the client cool
☐ to protect the client's hair from products
☐ to keep your brushes clean

7. What is the purpose of a visual study?

☐ to find out face shape
☐ to find out hair colour
☐ to work out the client's age

8. What are redness, swelling, itching and tightness a sign of?

☐ hayfever
☐ asthma
☐ allergy

9. What is a contra-indication?

☐ an allergy
☐ a funny face
☐ a reason not to treat

10. What is a contour brush used for?

☐ to shade and highlight the cheeks and face when doing corrective make-up
☐ to apply face powder
☐ to apply blusher

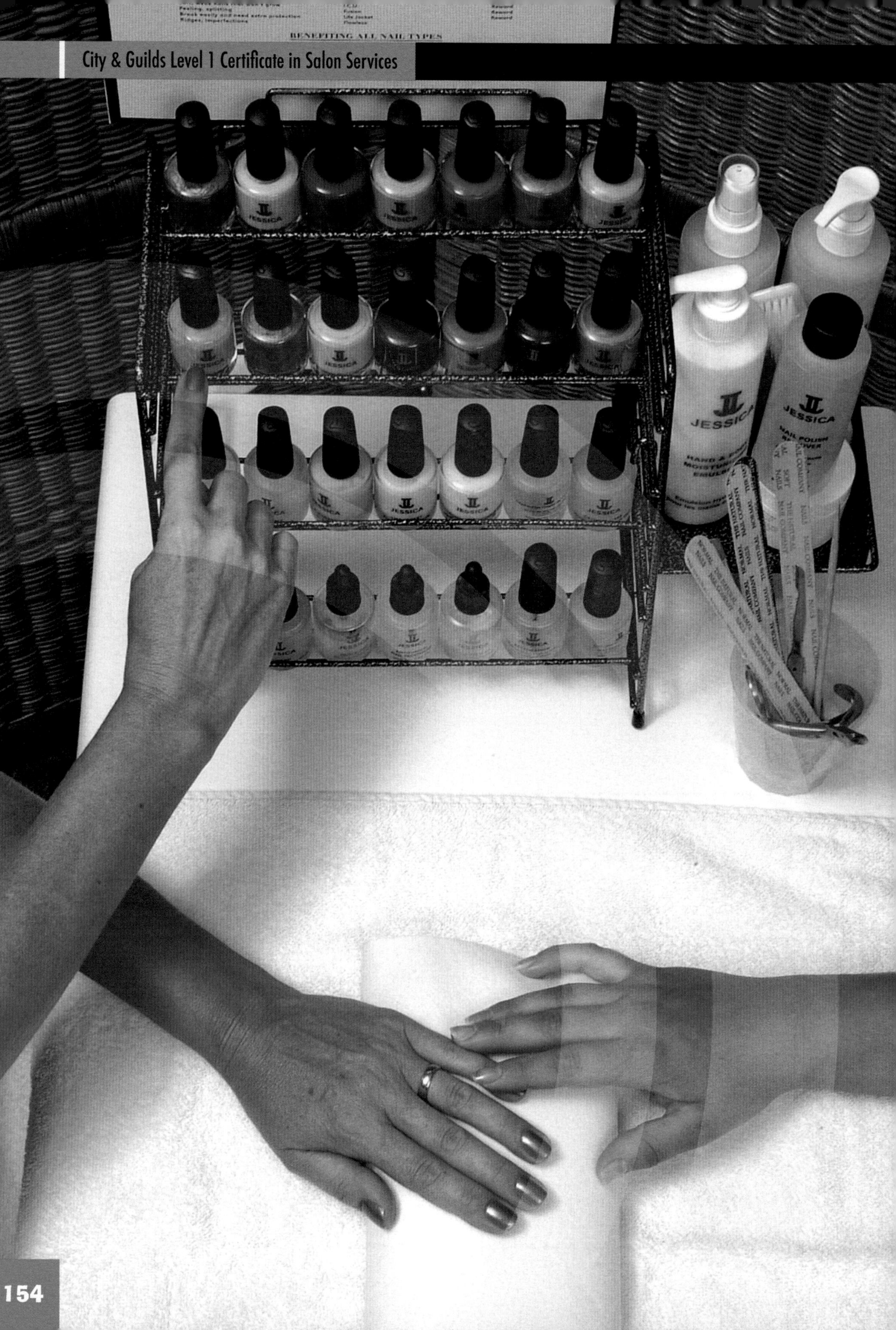
BENEFITING ALL NAIL TYPES
JESSICA

Unit 8

Basic manicure

Pampered nails are a real confidence booster! When a client looks at her nails after a manicure she will notice a big improvement. Even if she cares well for them herself, a professional manicure is a treatment worth having, and the client will be proud to show off her nails. From catwalk to high street, funky nail art designs to natural neutrals, nails are big business.

In this unit you will learn about:

- Why we manicure nails.
- The structure of the nail.
- Preparing for a manicure.
- When not to carry out a manicure.
- Products, materials and equipment.
- Carrying out a manicure.
- Creating a nail art design.

Towards the end of the course, you will be observed and assessed on:

- Setting up your work area.
- Carrying out a basic manicure.
- Tidying up after the treatment.

Why we manicure nails

A manicure is a treatment carried out to improve the condition of the hands and nails and to make them look more attractive. It includes cleaning and shaping the nails, care of the cuticles, hand massage and painting the nails with varnish.

TRY IT OUT!

Think of some reasons why a client might want a manicure. Here are a couple of examples to get you started:

- For a wedding day.
- To help stop nail biting.

The structure of the nail

The nail is made up of the following parts:

- The nail plate is the main part of the nail. It is hard, rectangular and curved. It covers and protects the nail bed and fingertip and is pink in colour.
- The free edge is the hardest part of the nail. It grows past the end of the nail bed and fingertip and is white in colour.
- The nail wall is the deep ridge that runs along the back and sides of the nail. It helps to stop germs entering the nail bed.
- The cuticle is found at the base of the nail. It protects the growing nail from germs.

When healthy, a nail should be pink, smooth and flexible with a white free edge which shows no signs of flaking or splitting. The cuticle should not be dry, rough or inflamed.

nail bed: skin beneath the nail

flexible: able to bend

inflamed: red and swollen

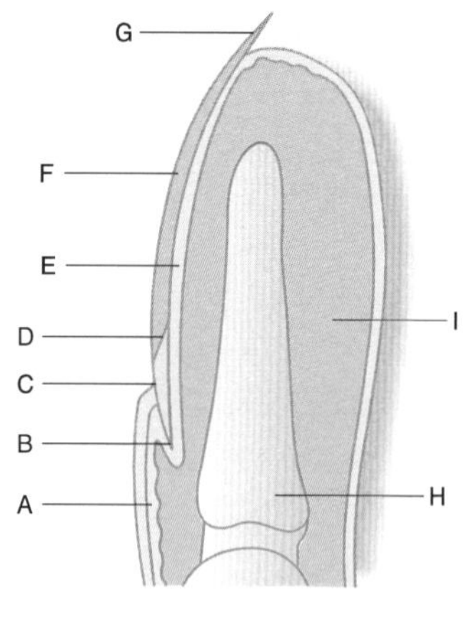

A nail wall
B matrix
C cuticle
D half moon (lanula)
E nail bed
F nail plate
G free edge
H bone
I subcutaneous tissue

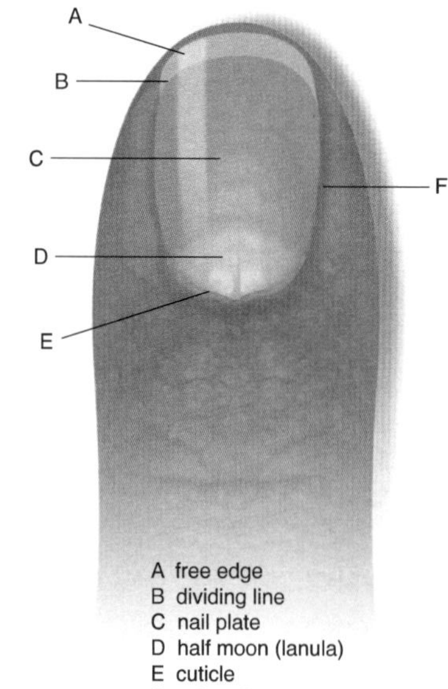

The parts of the nail

Nail shapes

Nail shapes will vary from one client to another. The natural shape usually mirrors the line of the cuticle and may be oval, rounded or square.

Oval

This shape softens the look of the hands and can make the fingers appear longer. It is quite hard-wearing because of its smooth edges.

Round

This shape is hard-wearing, strong and neat. However, it is not very flattering as it does not help to make the fingers look longer.

Square

This is a very good shape if the nails are fairly short and the fingers quite long. It does not look good on short fingers as it can make them appear even shorter. This shape of nail is less likely to break because the sides of the nails are supported by the nail wall.

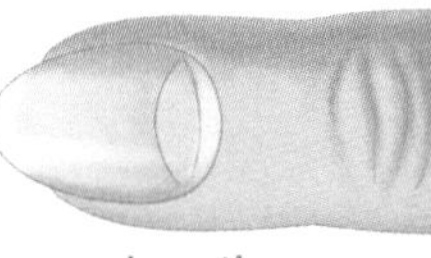
oval nail

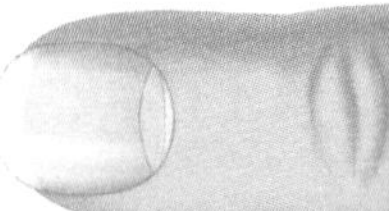
round nail

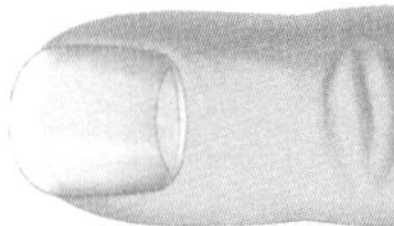
square nail

Nail shapes

OVER TO YOU...

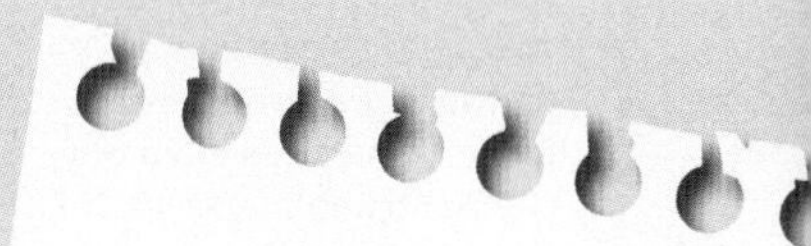

Look at the different nail shapes on your fellow students. Which are the most common?

Find pictures of various nail shapes. They could be from magazines, sketches or photographs. Add them to your portfolio or scrapbook, together with examples of false nail tips.

TRY IT OUT!

Briefly describe how you think your own hands and nails look so that a client will feel confident that you know what you are doing.

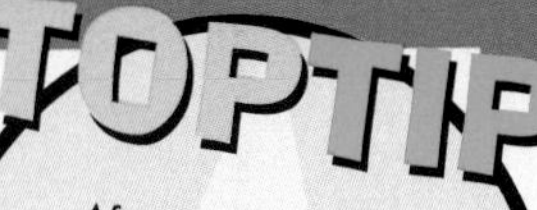

TOPTIP

After the treatment, note down on the record card the type of manicure you carried out, the products used and any advice you gave.

Preparing for a manicure

Before starting the manicure, you will need to carry out a client consultation. All information you find out must be written down on the client's record card before any part of the treatment is done. The record card should include:

- Information about the client's lifestyle and job – this will tell you about how the client's nails are treated and what to expect.
- Why the client wishes to have a manicure – this will tell you what the client would like to have done.
- The results of your visual study of the client's hands and nails – this will tell you the condition of the hands and nails.
- Any allergies.
- Any contra-indications.

contra-indications: reasons why you cannot treat the client

Visual study of the hands and nails

As part of the client consultation, you will need to look carefully at the condition of the client's hands and nails. This involves studying the texture and condition of the skin and nails. Follow the visual study procedures below to help you check the hands, nails and skin around the nails.

the way the surface looks and feels

Tell the senior therapist or your tutor if you notice anything unusual when carrying out a visual study of the hands and nails as it may be unsafe to carry out a treatment.

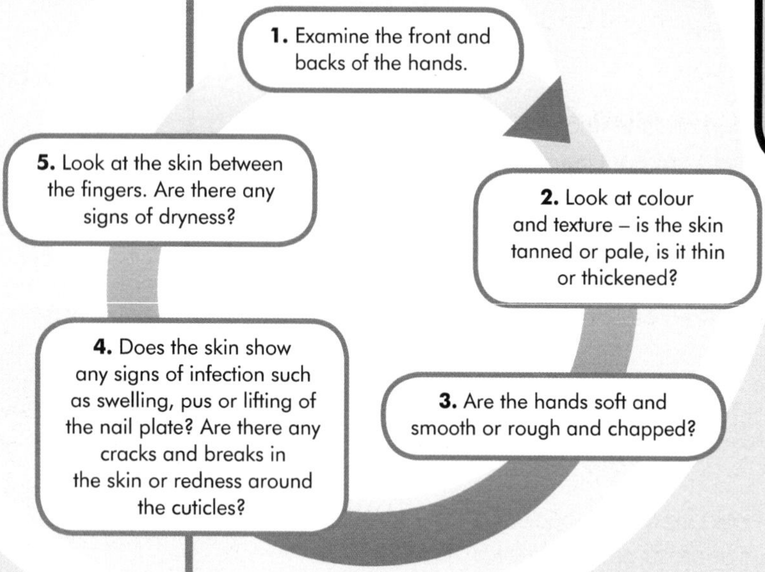

1. Examine the front and backs of the hands.

2. Look at colour and texture – is the skin tanned or pale, is it thin or thickened?

3. Are the hands soft and smooth or rough and chapped?

4. Does the skin show any signs of infection such as swelling, pus or lifting of the nail plate? Are there any cracks and breaks in the skin or redness around the cuticles?

5. Look at the skin between the fingers. Are there any signs of dryness?

Visual study of the hands

1. What shape are the nails?

2. What length are the nails? Have they been bitten?

3. Are the nails healthy, strong, pink, shiny and flexible or yellow, brittle, weak, thin?

4. Do the nails show any signs of nail diseases or disorders?

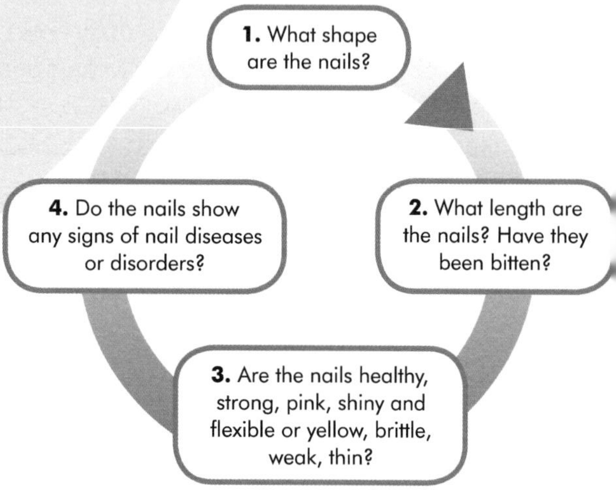

Visual study of the nails

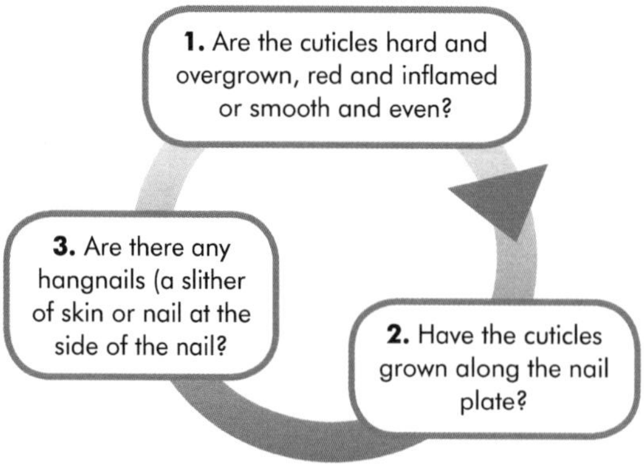

1. Are the cuticles hard and overgrown, red and inflamed or smooth and even?

2. Have the cuticles grown along the nail plate?

3. Are there any hangnails (a slither of skin or nail at the side of the nail?

Visual study of the skin around the nails

TOPTIP

Copy out each of the visual studies above onto a piece of A4 plain paper and laminate it. You can then keep this checklist by your side when you are carrying out your visual study of the hands and nails.

When not to carry out a manicure

You must never treat a client with any of the following contra-indications:

- Cuts or abrasions on or around the nail.
- Bruising or swelling around the nail.
- Severe nail damage.

scrapes or grazes

To make sure that you do not treat a client with a contra-indication ask yourself:

- Is there any redness, swelling, flaking or yellowing?
- If so, could this be a sign of a skin or nail disorder or an infection?

If you are unsure, you will need to ask a senior member of staff or your tutor whether:

- You can work around the condition.
- There is a total contra-indication and the client must not have the manicure.
- You can treat the client if he or she has a doctor's permission.

medical problem

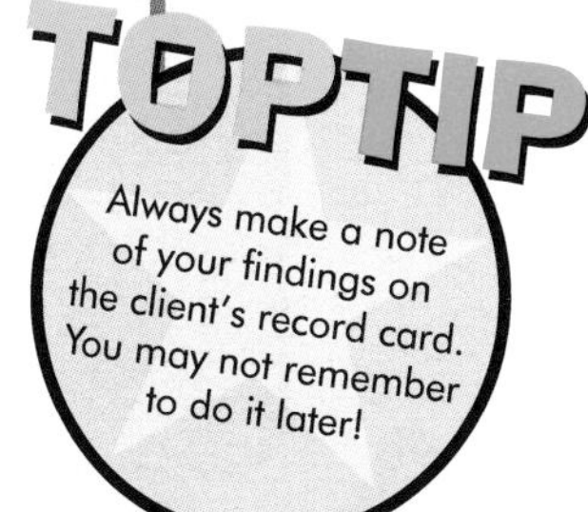

TOPTIP
Always make a note of your findings on the client's record card. You may not remember to do it later!

Checking for allergies

There may be ingredients in some manicure products that could cause clients to have an allergic reaction (when they itch or sneeze, or their skin reddens and might even swell). A very bad reaction might mean the client has to go to hospital. It is important that you check with the client whether they have any known allergies before you start the treatment.

If the client does have a reaction during the manicure, you must stop the treatment at once and remove all trace of the product from the client's skin with clean water. You should always report what happened to a senior member of staff.

Products, materials and equipment

Just before the treatment, set up your manicure tray with all the tools, equipment and products that you will need. Cover the tray with fresh couch roll and put on it:

- Sterilised tools in a jar filled with antiseptic.
- Emery boards (nail files).
- Two cotton wool covered orange sticks.
- Cotton wool and tissues.
- Manicure bowl filled with warm, soapy water.
- A selection of products including nail varnish remover, cuticle cream, moisturiser or massage cream and a range of varnish colours.
- A bowl for the client's jewellery.
- A record card for writing down the results of the visual study and consultation.

You will also need to have some clean towels and a gown nearby.

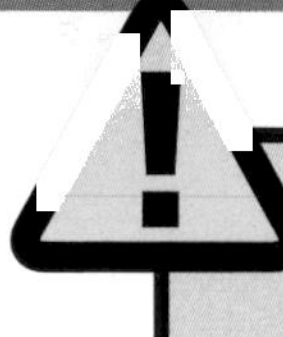

Always use clean water and clean towels for each new client so that you don't pass skin infections or nail diseases from client to client.

salon scene

Jemima started to prepare her work area for her client, but realised that she had forgotten all her tools, so she asked her friend Jazz if she could share. Jazz said yes but was a bit annoyed because Jemima was always forgetting her things and their tutor had said that they should not borrow each other's equipment. Jemima set up as best she could and started the treatment. It went well, she thought, because every time she needed something she simply called over to Jazz or went over to Jazz's manicure tray to get it. Unfortunately, her client seemed to be in a bad mood – she kept tutting throughout the treatment.

How do you think that Jemima's client felt during her treatment?

Was Jemima's behaviour professional? Explain your reasons.

Do you think that Jemima is being fair to Jazz? Explain your reasons

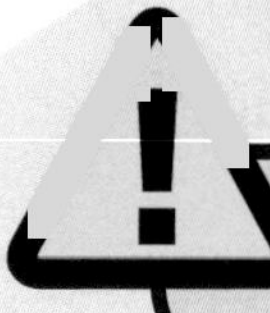

If you are right-handed, place the manicure tray to your right, if you are left-handed, set up on the left.

Products used during a manicure

Product	Type	Uses
Nail varnish remover	Liquid	Dissolves varnish so that it can be wiped easily off the nail plate with a piece of cotton wool.
Cuticle cream	Thick moisturising cream	Softens and nourishes the cuticle to make it easier to push back during a manicure without the skin splitting or pulling.
Moisturiser or cream	Rich cream	Massage into the hands and arms to soften the skin and relax the client.

feeds

Always follow the manufacturer's instructions when using manicure products. These will give you information on:

- How to use the product.
- How long to leave it on the skin.
- How to store it.
- How to use it safely.

Manicure materials

Materials	Uses
Cotton wool (small balls)	Soaked in nail varnish remover for taking off varnish – a clean piece of cotton wool is used for each nail. Wrapped around the tip of an orange stick for cuticle work, applying cuticle cream and nail cleaning.
Tissues	Used to wipe products from the nail. Tucked into the bottom of the client's sleeves to protect them from creams.
Towels	For drying hands and fingers after they have been soaked in water during the manicure.
Manicure bowl	A specially shaped gripper bowl that has a small hole in it for the thumb and a larger hole for fingers. It has a removable lid so that it can be cleaned inside properly after every client. It is filled with warm, soapy water to soak the client's hands during the manicure.
Hand soak	A mild soap which is mixed with warm water in the bowl. The warm, soapy water softens and cleans the nails and cuticles.
Dish	A small plastic or metal dish for the client's jewellery.
Waste bin or container	For waste disposal. A bin with a lid on is best.
Manicure cushion	For client comfort – the client's hands and wrists rest on this during the manicure.
Sterilising jar	For storing small metal tools during the treatment. The jar is filled with antiseptic or disinfectant solution.

Manicure tools

Tool	Uses
Spatula	For scooping out cream or lotion from pots.
Emery board/nail file	For filing and shaping. Emery boards come in different sizes and widths. The fine side is used for fingernails and the coarse side for male manicures and toenails as they tend to be thicker than the fingernails. (Dispose of after use for hygiene reasons.)
Orange stick	Both ends are coated in cotton wool for hygiene as the cotton wool can be removed and replaced when it has been used. The cotton wool softens the tip which prevents the cuticles and skin becoming sore during treatment. The pointed end is used for cleaning under the free edge and the hoof end is used for cuticle work.

Always use a spatula to scoop cream or lotion from a pot. It is unhygienic to use your fingers.

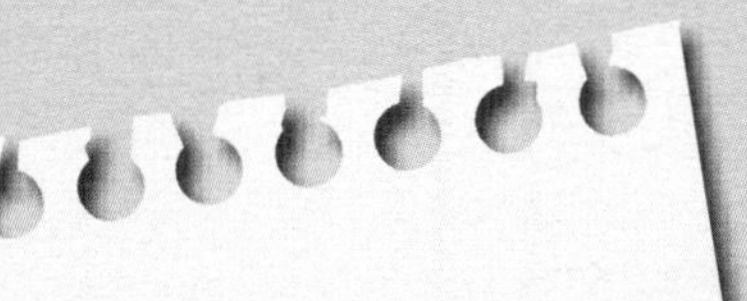

OVER TO YOU...

Find pictures of manicure products and equipment. They could be from magazines, sketches or photographs. Add them to your portfolio or scrapbook.

TRY IT OUT!

Pair up with a classmate. Set up a manicure tray with all the tools, materials and products. Look at it for one minute, then cover the tray and list all the items on it. How many did you remember?

Carrying out a manicure

A manicure is a sequence of mini treatments which are aimed to improve the look and condition of the hands and nails. A complete manicure should take about 30–45 minutes. Follow this step-by-step to complete a professional nail treatment.

> Before starting the manicure, check that both you and your client are comfortable. Pay particular attention to your posture. If the back is overstretched from reaching in order to carry out the treatment, it will cause back pain, neck ache and tiredness.

How to carry out a manicure

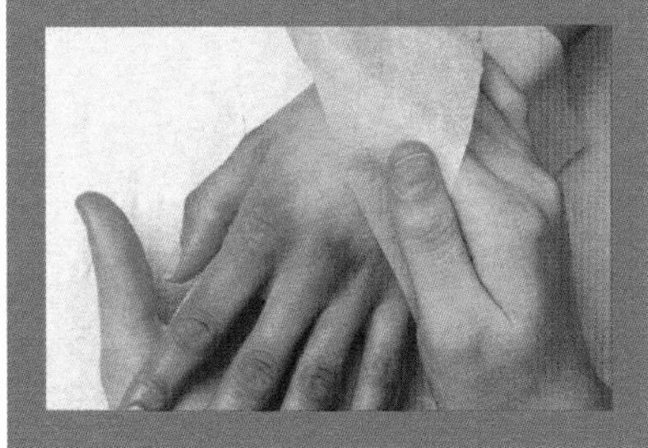

1 Wipe over the front and back of the client's hands with antiseptic.

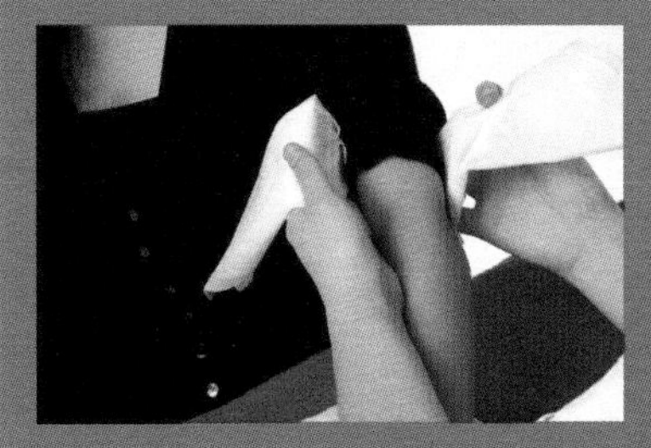

2 Roll the client's sleeves up to the elbow, then tuck tissue around them for protection against creams and lotions.

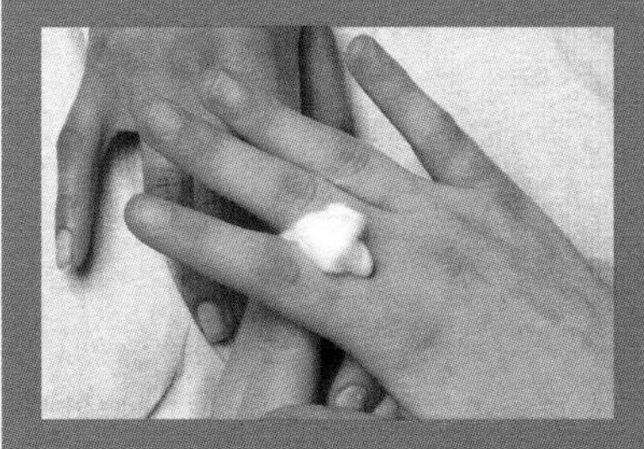

3 Right hand. Soak cotton wool with nail varnish remover, then place between two fingers. Hold onto the nail plate for a few seconds, then wipe downwards to remove the varnish.

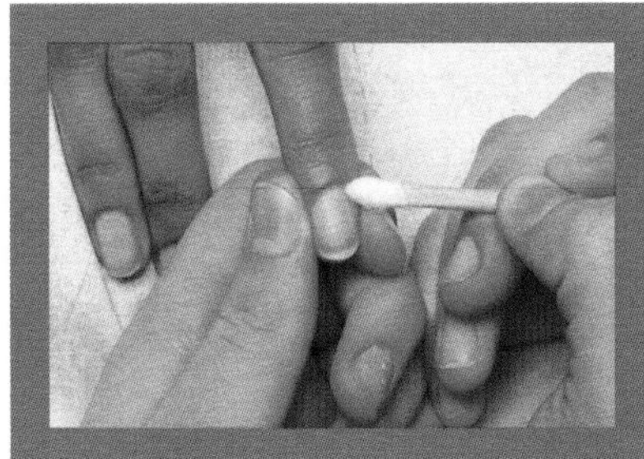

4 Right hand. Cover an orange stick with cotton wool, then dip the end into some nail varnish remover. Use this to go round the cuticle, where dark or bright varnish tends to stain.

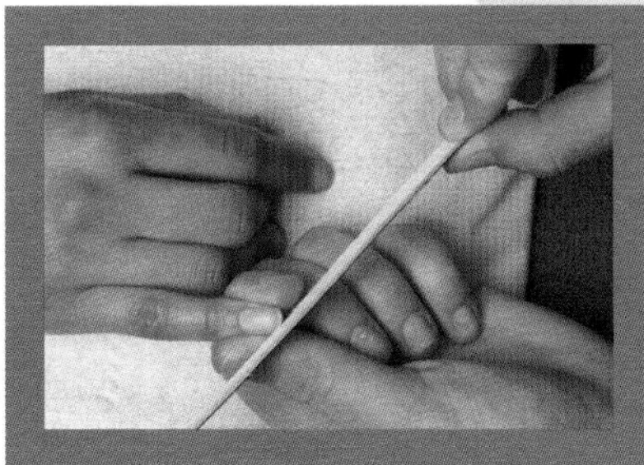

5 File the nails on the right hand using the fine side of the emery board. (See The right way to file nails on page 165.)

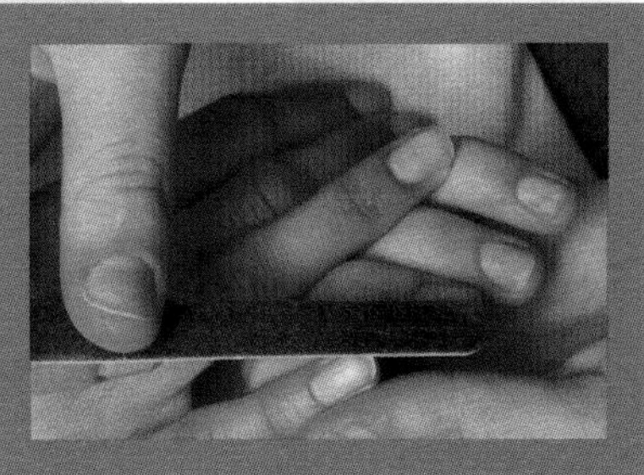

6 Right hand. Turn the emery board lengthways to the nail and very gently buff the tip of the nail with the fine side.

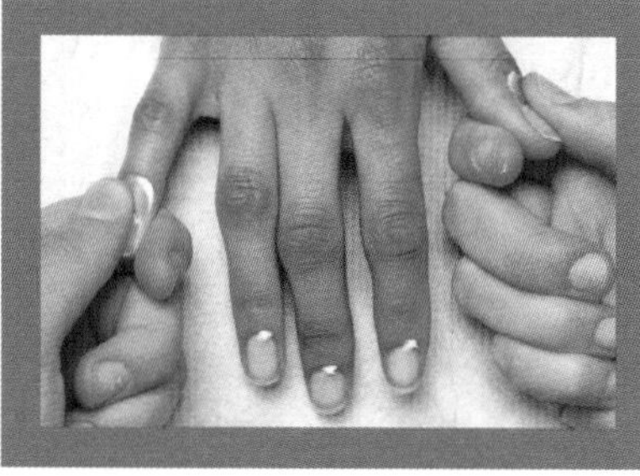

7 Right hand. Use a clean spatula to scoop out a small (pea-sized) amount of cuticle cream. Next, dip a covered orange stick into the cream and apply it to the centre of the cuticles on each nail. Massage in the cuticle cream in a circular action, so that it covers the nail and cuticles.

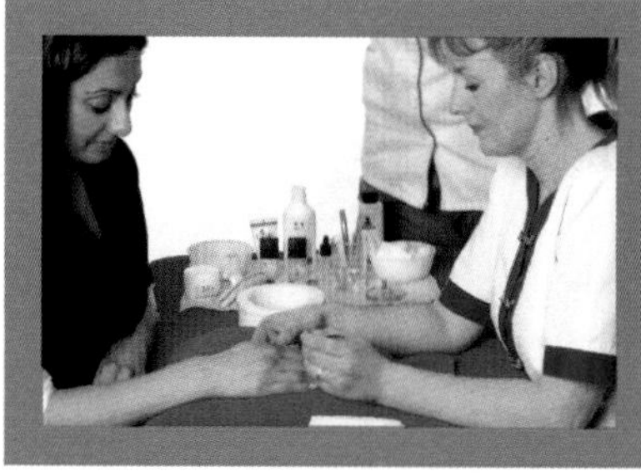

8 Place the client's right hand in the manicure bowl containing warm, soapy water. Repeat steps 3–7 on the client's left hand.

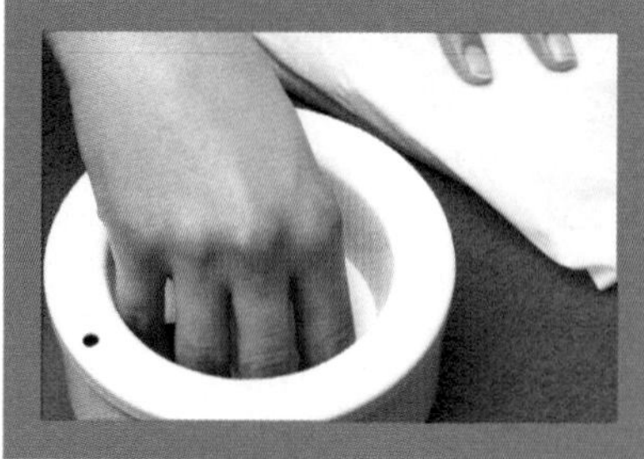

9 Take the client's right hand out of the water. Place the client's left hand in the water.

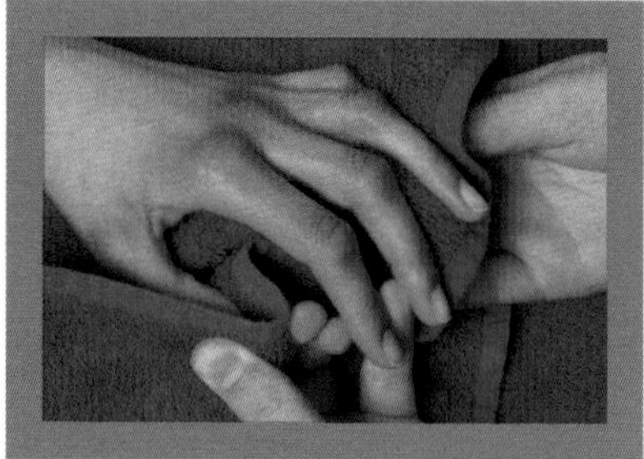

10 Dry the client's right hand and nails thoroughly using a towel, pushing the cuticles back with the towel as you go.

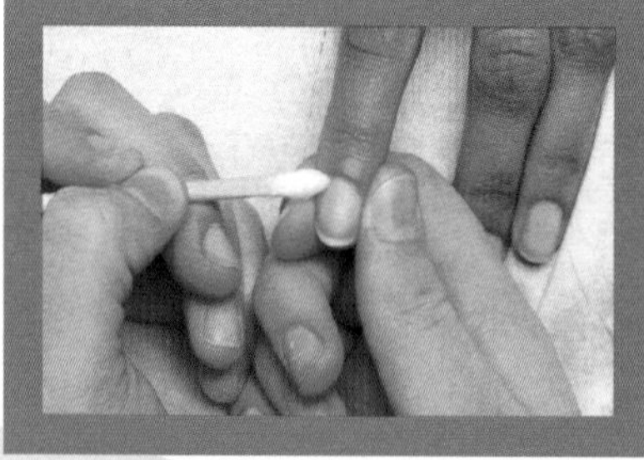

11 On the right hand, the senior therapist may do further cuticle work using cuticle remover.

12 Repeat steps 10 and 11 on the client's left hand.

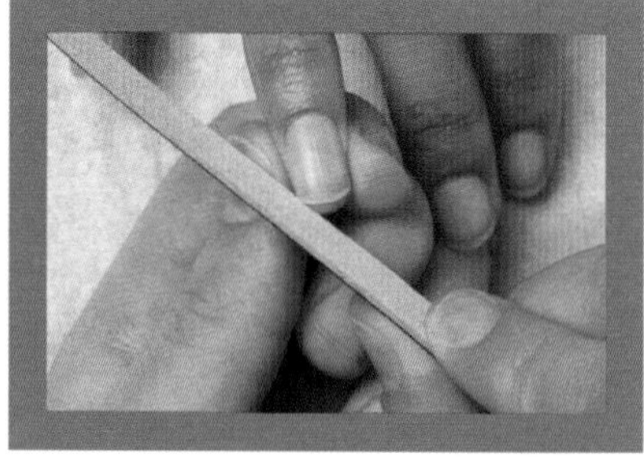

13 Tidy up the free edges of the nails on both hands with the emery board, as fine wisps of nail may have appeared.

14 Carry out a hand and arm massage.

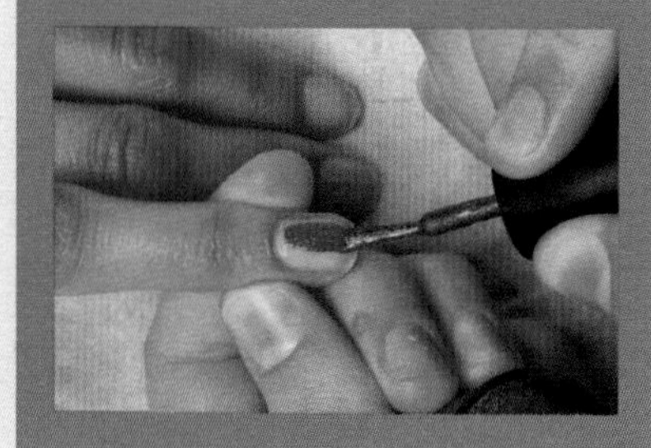

15 Go over the nails with nail varnish remover to de-grease them, as you did at the start of the manicure (step 3). Paint the nails, following the routine described on page 167.

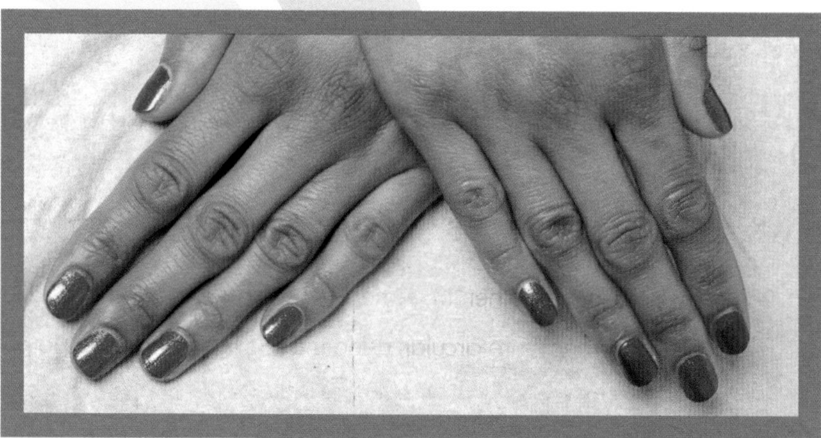

16 The finished result.

The right way to file nails

File the nails using the fine side of the emery board. Do not saw in both directions, as this will cause the nail to split. Use the file at a 45-degree angle to the nail and a side to centre action.

Turn the emery board lengthways to the nail and very gently buff the tip of the nail with the fine side – this is called bevelling and is done to seal the free edges against splitting and peeling back.

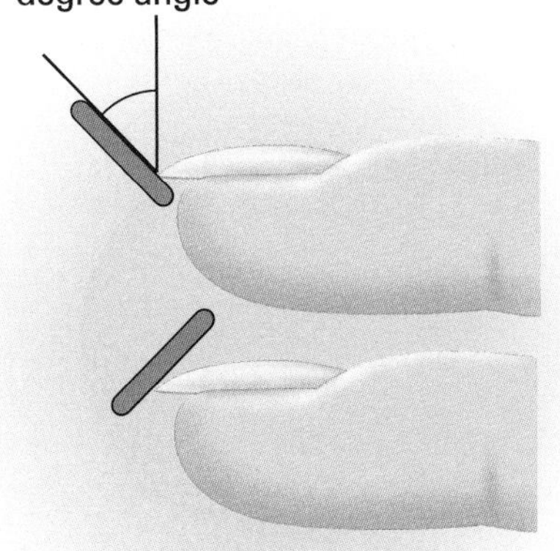

Use the file at a 45-degree angle

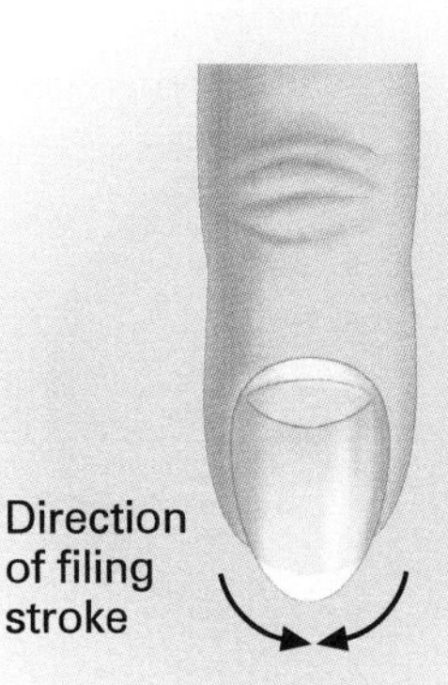

File the nail using a side to centre action

If there are any hangnails or loose bits of skin on the cuticles, tell the senior therapist or your tutor, who will remove them.

When shaping the nails you will need to think about:

- The shape of the nail before treatment – you can only improve the natural shape of the nail, not change it.
- The client's lifestyle and job, e.g. long nails may not be suitable for a client who plays sport.
- The client's wishes.
- The shape of the cuticles – for a natural look, follow the curve of the cuticle with the same nail shape.

Massage and moisturise

Moisturising softens and smoothes the skin and is a perfect finish to a manicure. The moisturiser or massage cream is applied and rubbed into the skin using rubbing and kneading movements, known as massage. Massage is relaxing and helps the client feel good.

There are three main massage movements:

- Effleurage is a gentle stroking movement. It is used at the beginning or end of a treatment or to join up other movements. It has a soothing and relaxing effect.
- Petrissage movements are circular, using the thumbs or fingertips to put pressure on the muscles.
- Tapotement is a more stimulating movement and uses the fingers to produce light tapping and quick pinching or gentle slapping movements.

For the Level 1 Certificate in Salon Services, it is not necessary for you to follow a set massage routine using all the movements. However, it is important to carry out some sort of routine that is relaxing to the client. For example, start with lighter strokes which become deeper. Start with the arm (up to the elbow), then move down to the hands and then the fingers.

How to do a hand massage

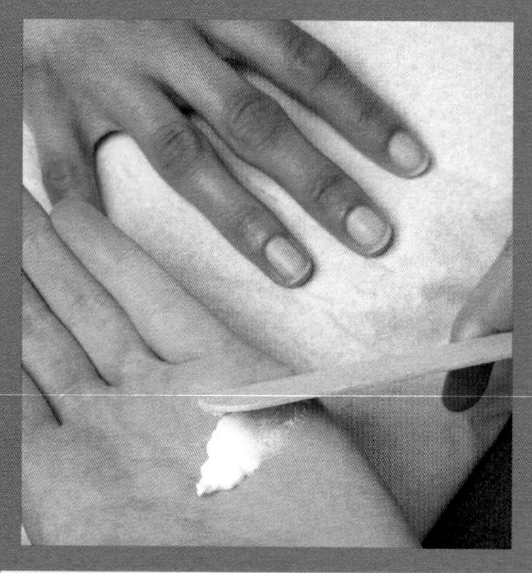

1 Using a spatula, place a small amount of massage cream or moisturiser into the palm of your hands.

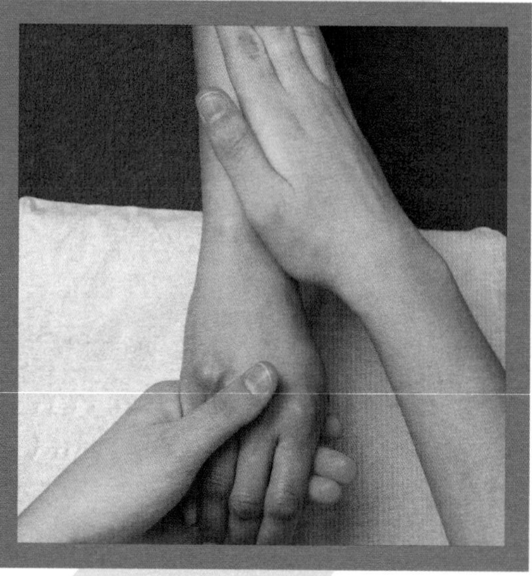

2 Stroke the cream onto the skin of the client's arms using smooth upward effleurage movements.

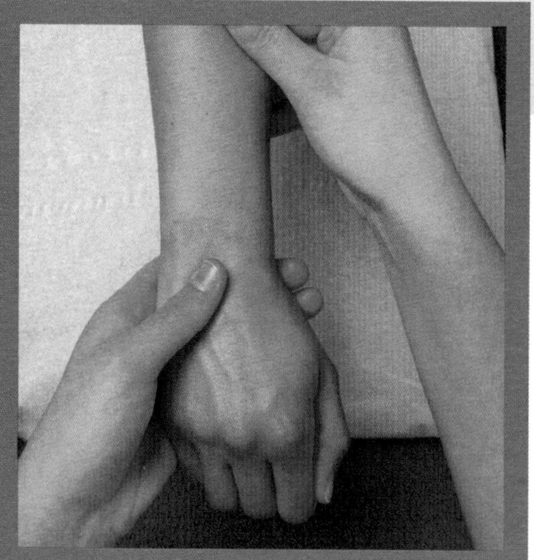

3 Massage using a variety of flowing effleurage and gentle kneading (petrissage) movements.

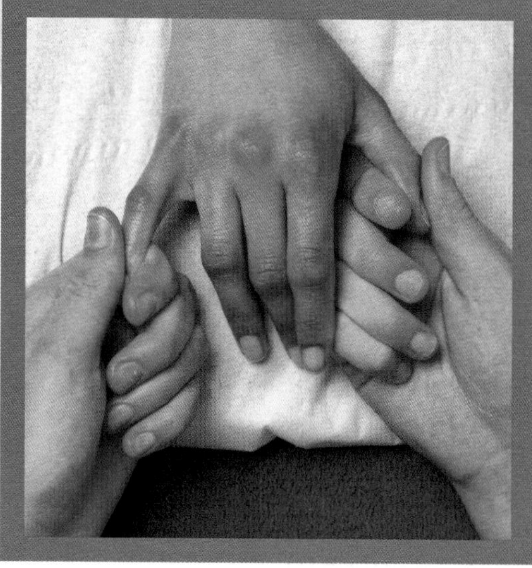

4 Use petrissage techniques on the fingers of both hands.

Paint and polish

Paint or polish completes the look. Before you paint her nails, ask the client to put her jewellery back on, put on her jacket or coat and take out her car keys. The natural hardening time of varnish can be up to two hours. Even if the nails feel dry to touch, they can still dent if knocked. After this, show the client the colour range and ask her to choose one.

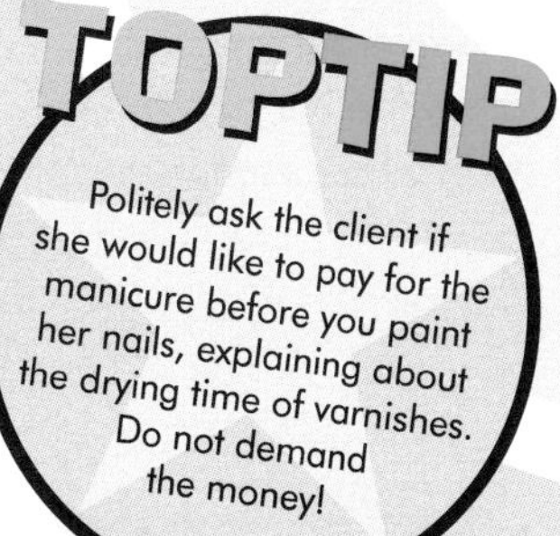

Politely ask the client if she would like to pay for the manicure before you paint her nails, explaining about the drying time of varnishes. Do not demand the money!

OVER TO YOU...

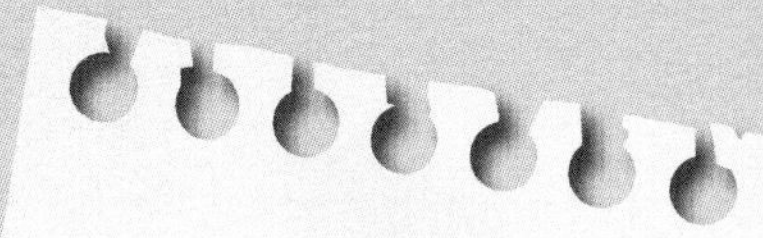

Find pictures of nail varnish colours. They could be from magazines, sketches or photographs. Add them to your portfolio or scrapbook.

About nail polishes

Base coats can be clear or pale coloured. They are applied to the nail plate before varnish to:

- Smooth the nail.
- Cut down on staining from dark and bright coloured varnishes.
- Help prevent early chipping or wearing off of the colour.

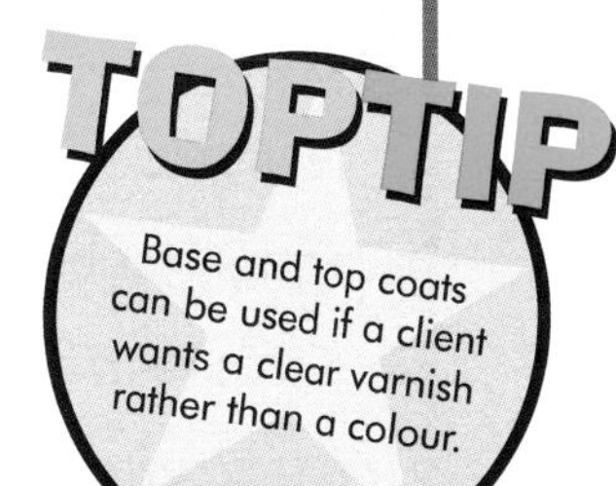

Base and top coats can be used if a client wants a clear varnish rather than a colour.

Top coats are usually clear and are used to:

- Give a high shine to the coloured nails.
- Help make the varnish last longer.

Nail hardeners are like clear varnishes but contain extra ingredients to provide the nails with a tough coating.

Nail strengtheners are usually clear and contain nourishing and strengthening ingredients to help weak nails grow.

Cream nail varnish is good for nails with a lot of ridges and dents as it does not show them up.

Pearlised nail varnish contains ingredients which give the polish a shimmery look. It is best used on nails in good condition as it shows up ridges and dents.

Painting the client's nails

Nail varnish should be painted on in a methodical way. Look at the diagram which will show you how. Begin with one central application (1), then apply the varnish to the right (2) and the left (3) of the nail. Finally, go over the whole nail to smooth the varnish (4).

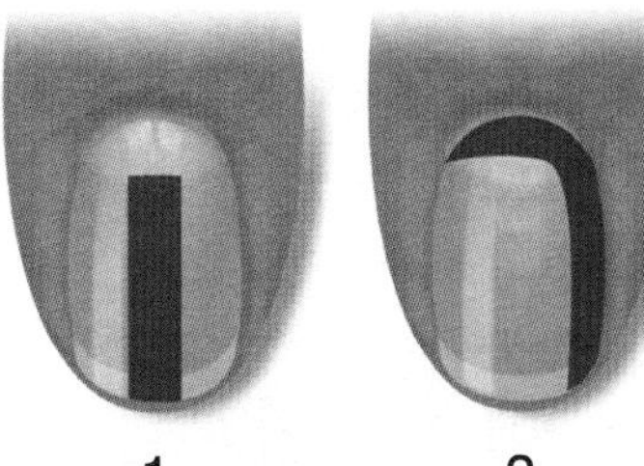

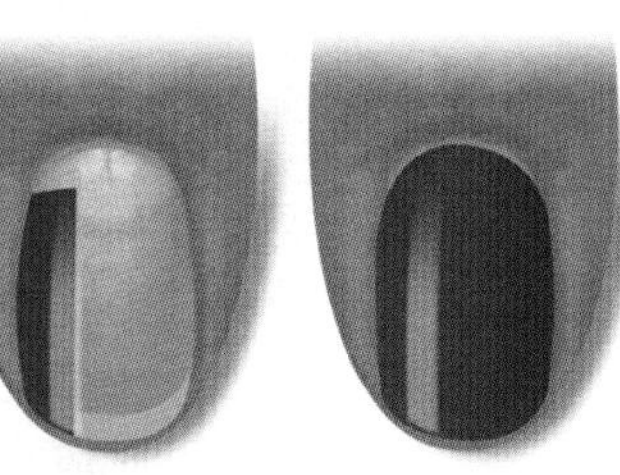

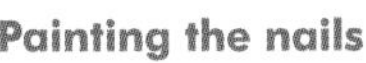
Painting the nails

methodical: careful and organised

To prevent smudging, follow the finger rotation method of painting.

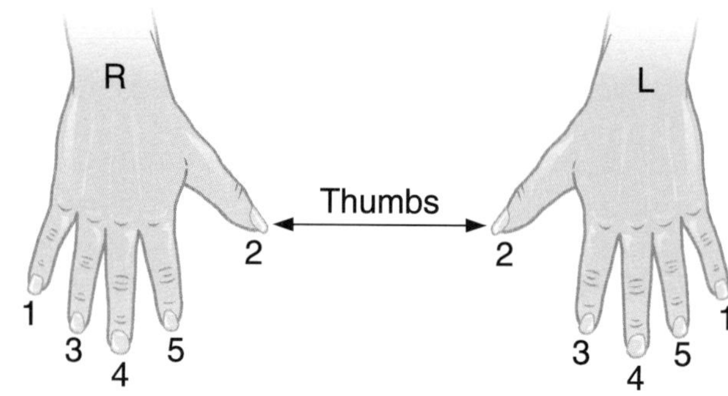

The finger rotation method of painting

Dear Nat

I really enjoy painting nails, but the other day I made a mistake and needed to clean up around the nail. I tried using a cotton wool bud but ended up smudging the whole lot! The client didn't look too pleased. What should I have done?

From Agnessa

Nat says

If you get varnish on the cuticles, it's best to clean it off straight away. Wet nail varnish is easier to remove than dry, so don't wait until the end of the painting to clean around the nail. Have ready a cotton wool covered orange stick (pointed end) which has been soaked in nail varnish remover.

Nail painting tips

Do	Don't
Make sure that you have enough varnish on the brush to do a whole nail.	Overload the brush – paint will drip down and flood the nail with too much varnish.
Paint thinly and use only a few strokes.	Paint thickly as it will take too long to dry.
Leave a small gap at the base of the nail before the cuticle.	Use too many brush strokes as the finish will be lumpy and uneven.
Hold the bottle while you paint.	Paint right up to the cuticle – the varnish will seep into the skin and will look messy.

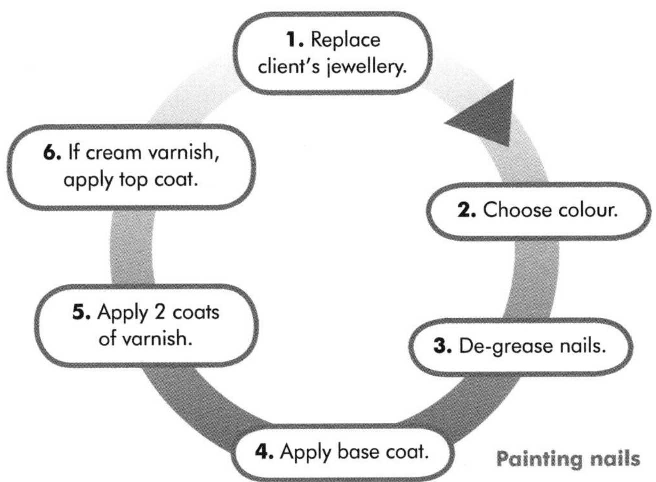
1. Replace client's jewellery.
2. Choose colour.
3. De-grease nails.
4. Apply base coat.
5. Apply 2 coats of varnish.
6. If cream varnish, apply top coat.

Painting nails

Choosing a nail polish

Nail varnish comes in many colours and you need to think about a few things first so that you can help the client choose the right colour:

The length of the nails

A very bright colour on short or bitten nails will only draw attention to them and make them look shorter than they are.

The condition of the cuticles

Red looking cuticles can look even worse if the nails are painted in a bright or pearlised varnish. Pale and neutral colours in a cream varnish will look better.

The client's home life and job

If a client has a job that could cause the nails to chip quickly, then it is best to choose a colour that is not going to show the odd little chip too much.

The client's skin colour

Orange, peach or beige colours show up the bluish colour in skin with poor circulation. Pinks clash with reddish skin tones.

The condition and smoothness of the nails

Pearlised varnish will show up any dents or ridges, so use a ridge filling base coat and a cream varnish.

The size of the fingernails

Dark colours make the nails look smaller.

The occasion

Is the client having her nails painted for a special occasion? If so, the type of occasion will help decide which colour or effect is required. For example, a bride will usually want a pale, natural or clear varnish colour, or one that matches the colour of her bouquet or bridesmaids' dresses. A client going to a party will probably want a much bolder, brighter colour.

salon scene

Mandy was getting ready for her first client. She prepared her manicure tray thoroughly and checked that her all her tools were sterilised and her work area was clean and tidy.

The manicure was going well and the client was very friendly. As Mandy started on the hand massage, Ushma, in the next work area, asked if she could borrow the nail varnish remover. Mandy stopped the massage and reached across to pass Ushma the bottle. As she did so, the bottle slipped out of her hands and landed on the floor, spilling nail varnish remover everywhere. In her panic, Mandy jumped up to try to catch the bottle and knocked the contents of the manicure tray over the client's clothes. The products spilled out over the client's skirt. Everything in the room went quiet. Mandy ran out of the room.

List everything that Mandy did wrong.

How could each disaster be avoided in the future?

What did Ushma do wrong?

Could Mandy have coped better with the situation?

Creating a nail art design

Nail art is great fun and gives you the chance to express yourself. Hand-painted nail art is quick and easy to apply and requires only a few supplies. The techniques are easy to learn and, with a little practice and effort, a stunning design can be achieved.

There are three main steps to a nail art treatment:

1. Apply a base coat.
2. Apply the design.
3. Seal with a top coat.

Designs can be painted on artificial nails or natural nails.

Nail art paints are usually water-based acrylic paints and come in many colours. They can be easily mixed to create more colours. Many different effects can be achieved with a selection of nail art brushes, dotting tools and marbling tools.

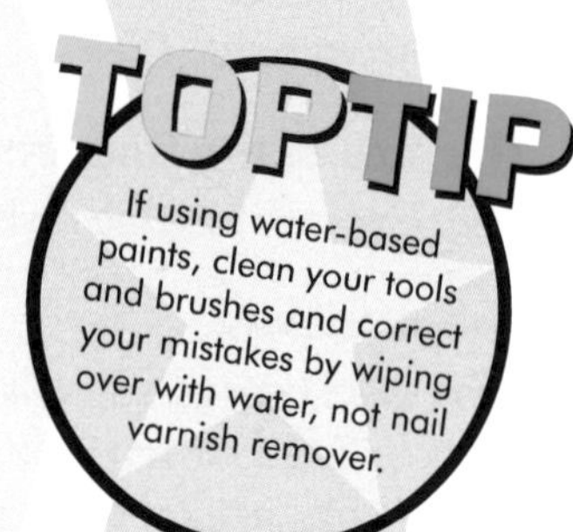

TOPTIP
If using water-based paints, clean your tools and brushes and correct your mistakes by wiping over with water, not nail varnish remover.

Nails should be painted with a base colour that will provide a smooth, coloured canvas on which the nail art will be painted. Nail varnish is usually used for the base. The base colour must be touch dry before starting your design.

Nail art products, tools and techniques

Foils

This is a very easy technique, as the foils already have the design on them. Simply apply foil adhesive to the nail. When the adhesive goes clear put the foil onto the nail and press down, gently remove the foil and the design will be on the nail. Finally, seal the design.

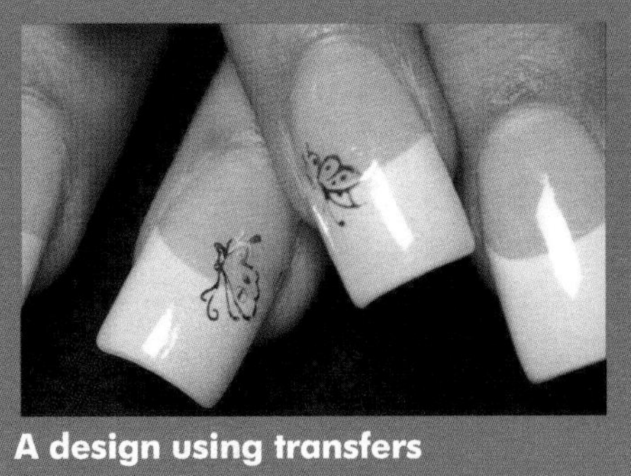
A design using transfers

Glitter

Glitter polish and glitter dust will bring your nail art alive. Polishes are applied directly onto the nail. The easiest way to apply glitter dust is to first coat the nail with sealer, then dip it into the dust. Another method is to sprinkle dust onto slightly wet varnish.

Transfers

There are two types of transfer:

- Sticky back – peel off the back and stick to the nail.
- Water decals – these are soaked off by applying a few drops of water to the transfer.

Gemstones and rhinestones

These come in many different shapes, sizes and colours. Use an orange stick tipped with a small ball of Blu-tack to pick up the gemstone or rhinestone and place it on the nail while the varnish is still tacky. Allow the polish to dry before applying sealer or topcoat.

TOPTIP

Advise clients to apply top coat every other day to prevent chipping.

Stencils

These provide an outline for a pattern or shape on the nail.

Fine liner brush

This is used to paint detail on the nail.

Striper brush

A very long, thin brush dipped in paint can achieve fine stripes, unusual patterns or marbling. Marbling can be done by creating dots with a special effects tool and then flicking the colour from side to side with the striper brush.

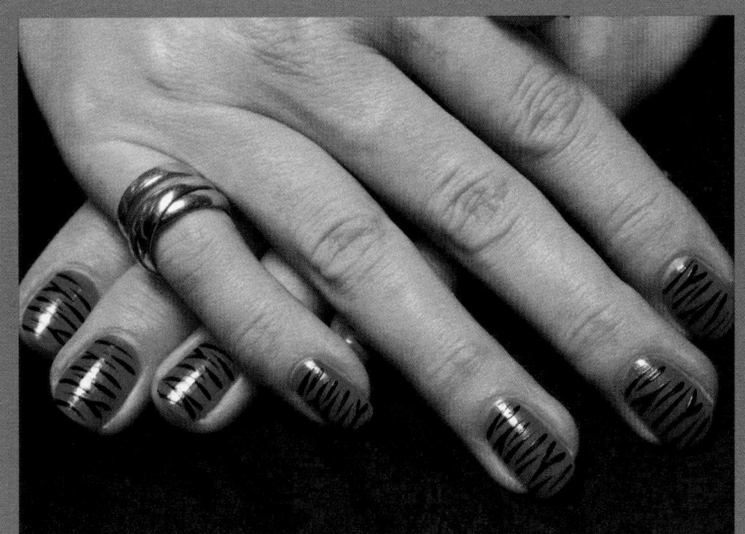
A design using a striper brush

Special effects (dotting) tool

This tool can be used to create dots and petals. Just dip the end into the acrylic paint and dot onto the nail.

1. Choose a varnish colour.
2. Remove the old varnish.
3. File the nails.
4. Push back the cuticles with a cotton wool covered orange stick.
5. Massage the hands with hand cream.
6. Remove grease from the nail plate.
7. Apply the base coat.
8. Carry out the nail art design.
9. Seal the design.
10. Give aftercare advice.

Nail art procedure

TOP TIP

Never add nail varnish remover to nail varnish to thin it out – it will only thin it out enough for one use and after this, it will thicken up even more than it was before.

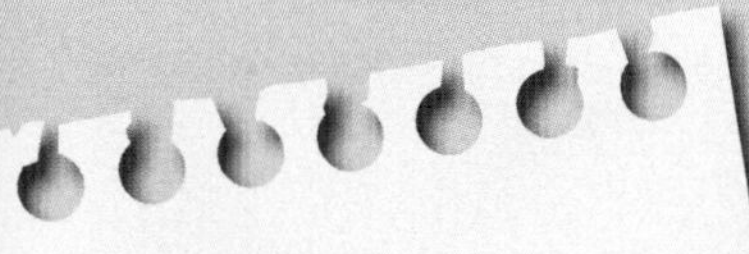

OVER TO YOU...

Find pictures of nail art designs. They could be from magazines, sketches or photographs. Add them to your portfolio or scrapbook.

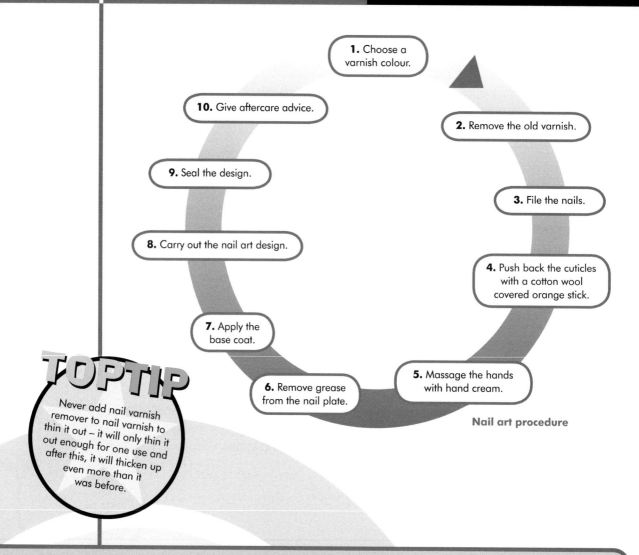

Check what you know...

1. What is a contra-indication?
- [ ] a type of record card
- [ ] a question and answer session between you and your client
- [ ] a condition that may mean you will not be able to treat

2. The nail wall is:
- [ ] the deep ridge that runs along the back and sides of the nail
- [ ] the growing part of the nail
- [ ] the white edge of the nail

3. What four things must be included on a client's record card?
- [ ] name, age, nail condition, whether or not they were a nice customer
- [ ] name, address, favourite colour, appointment details
- [ ] name, address, telephone number, treatment details

4. How do you decide on the shape and length of a client's nails?
- [ ] ask her what she would like
- [ ] follow the fashion
- [ ] do them square

5. What is the purpose of a manicure?
- [ ] to improve the condition of the skin, nails and cuticles
- [ ] to improve the condition of the skin, nails and nail varnish
- [ ] to stop the nails chipping

6. What is the procedure for a manicure?
- [ ] file, cuticle work, soak, massage, paint
- [ ] file, soak, cuticle work, massage, paint
- [ ] soak, file, cuticle work, massage, paint

7. What is the purpose of cuticle cream?
- [ ] to soften and nourish the cuticles
- [ ] to make the cuticles easier to cut
- [ ] to dissolve extra skin on the nail plate

8. What is the white edge of the nail called?
- [ ] the flexible edge
- [ ] the nail edge
- [ ] the free edge

9. How long should a manicure take to complete?
- [ ] 1 hour
- [ ] 25–30 minutes
- [ ] 30–45 minutes

10. Before applying a base coat:
- [ ] apply the top coat
- [ ] de-grease the nails
- [ ] apply nail art

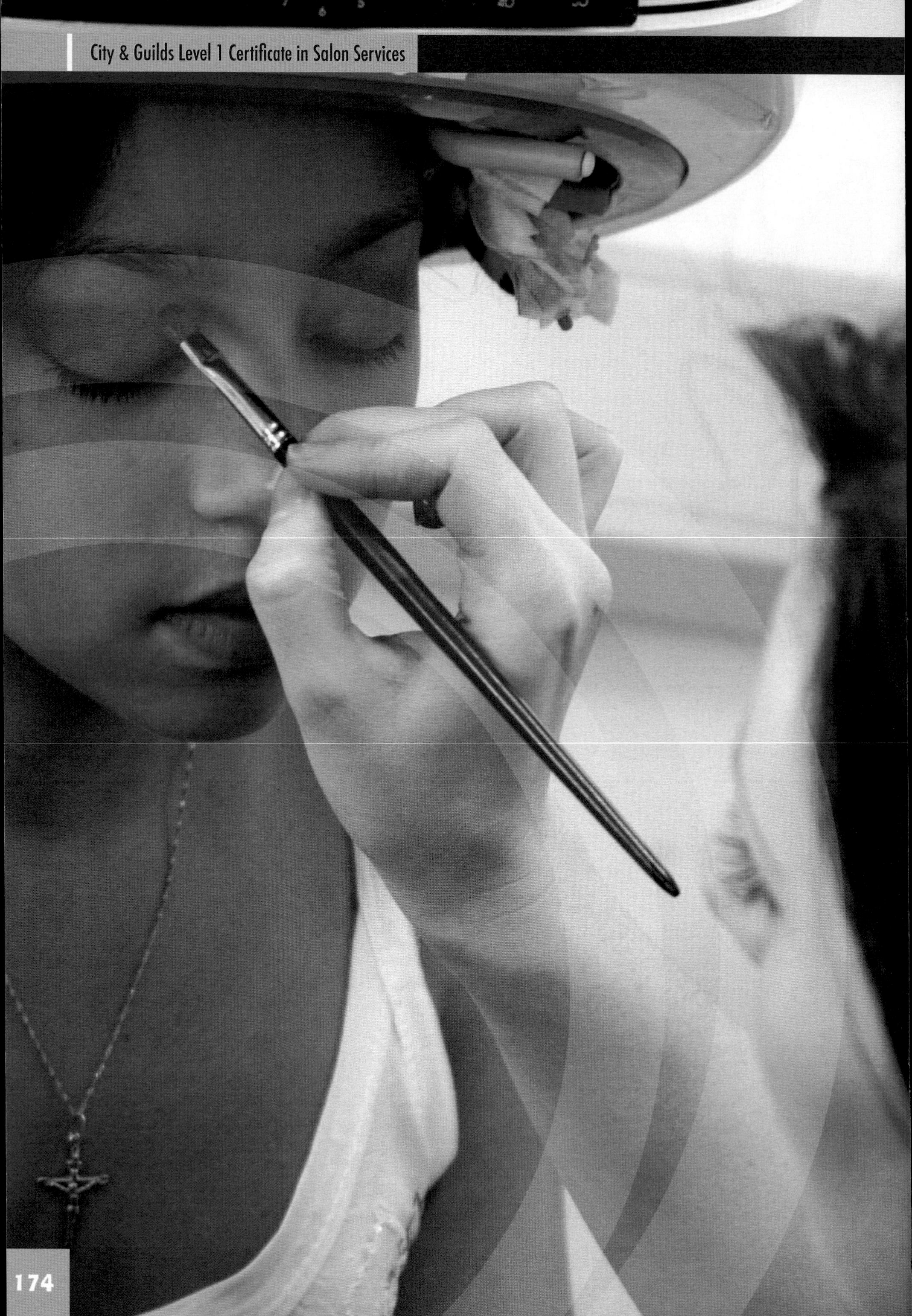

Unit 9

Working in hair and beauty

The hair and beauty industry offers so many different career opportunities. What other job offers you the chance to travel, have fun, meet exciting people and do something you love while also helping others to feel good about themselves? From working in a salon, being your own boss, to working on a cruise liner, hair and beauty can offer you all this and the chance to reach management level with a top salary to match!

Hair and beauty is a career that you can take with you, wherever your personal life goes. There will always be someone who will want their feet pedicured or hair cut into the latest style. It is no longer a luxury to have a wide range of hair and beauty treatments and services – they are all part of a busy person's lifestyle. If you are good at what you do, you will never be short of work. This unit will guide you through the different career paths you could take.

In this unit you will learn about:

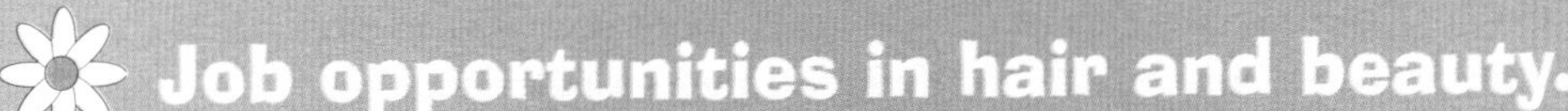

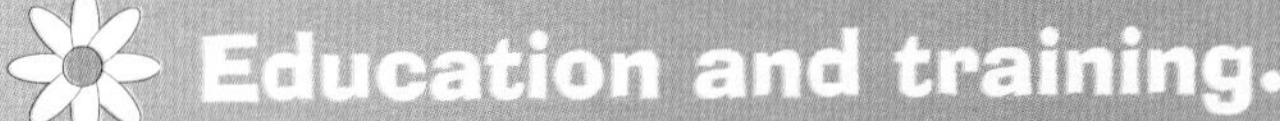

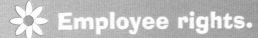

- Employee rights.

Job opportunities in hair and beauty

There is a dazzling range of job opportunities in the hair and beauty industry, from working in salons and nail bars to stylists on fashion photo shoots, from consultants in department stores to hair and make-up artists in television and theatre, or you might wish to teach and train others. Look at the job profiles over the following pages. They will give you an idea of the jobs that could one day be open to you!

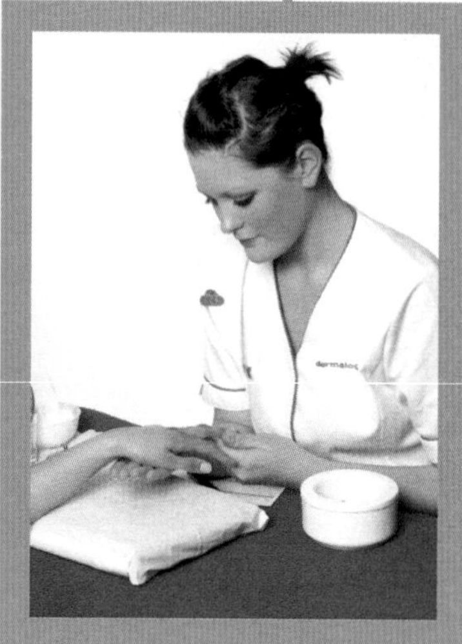

Nail technician

The job – Applying artificial nails to the surface of the natural nail. Skills needed are speed and attention to detail.

Training – S/NVQ Nail Services Levels 2 and 3.

Pay – A newly qualified nail technician can expect the national minimum wage (around £8,000 a year). An experienced technician may earn around £10,000 a year, while a highly experienced self-employed nail technician can earn over £25,000.

Hours – Tend to be set if working in a salon but self-employed work can be unsociable with long hours.

The good – Seeing clients leave the salon with beautiful nails.

The bad – Sitting for long periods leaning over a nail station (can cause neck and back ache). Some nail products have an overpowering odour.

Advice for students – After training, shadow an experienced nail technician for a couple of months, even if you are not paid!

shadow: follow a qualified person in order to watch and learn

Hair stylist

The job – Styling hair using a variety of techniques (cutting, colouring, perming, relaxing, braiding etc).

Training – A minimum of S/NVQ Level 2.

Pay – Starting salary is usually in the region of £10,000 a year. This can rise to £20,000 – £25,000. This doesn't include tips!

Hours – Days can be quite long and you will probably have to work some evenings. You will almost certainly have to work weekends, but you will get a day off in the week instead.

The good – Meeting lots of people and working in a creative and fashionable industry. There are also opportunities to travel, teach your skills to other people, work on photo shoots, style the rich and famous – the list is never ending!

The bad – The pay is not great to start with and you're on your feet most of the day. Working weekends and evenings is also a downside.

Advice for students – Work hard and get all the training that is offered to you. Start working in a salon as soon as possible – get a Saturday job so that you can get some hands-on experience and improve your people skills. This is also a good way to find out if hairdressing is the career for you. Most important of all, enjoy it!

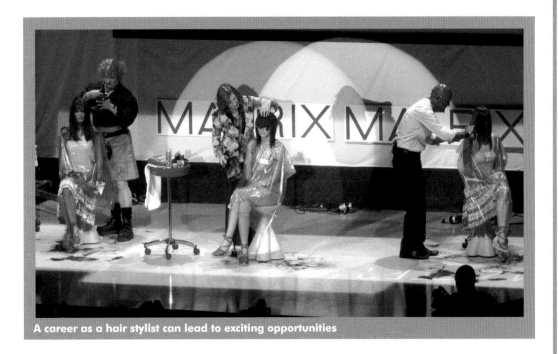

A career as a hair stylist can lead to exciting opportunities

Beauty therapist

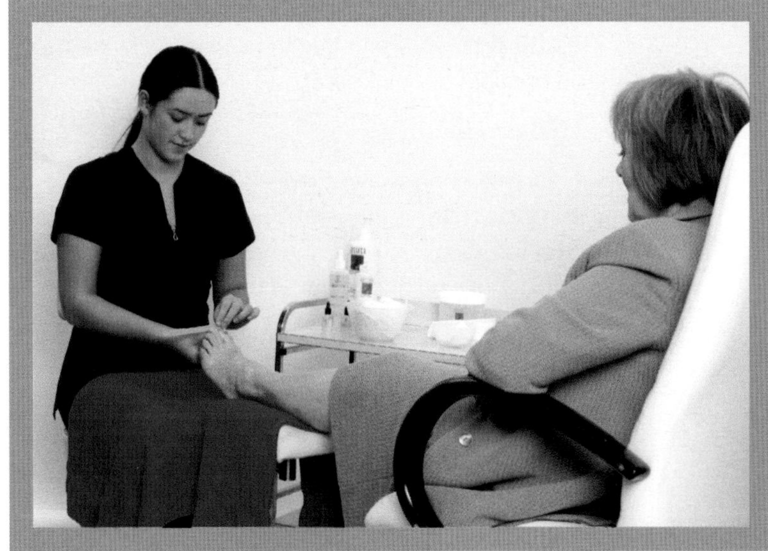

The job – Carrying out a wide range of beauty treatments, depending on level of qualification.

Training – Usually a full-time 1–2 year course at college leading to an S/NVQ Level 3. Other options include combined college and workplace training such as apprenticeships or shorter courses at private colleges.

Pay – Often low at the start, rising to an excellent wage for experienced therapists. Therapists who bring in a lot of money for the business may also receive commission.

Hours – Usually a 5-day week. For salons operating on a 6- or 7-day week, therapists work a rota system so that every member of staff takes a turn working unsociable hours, including late opening in the evenings.

The good – Carrying out a wide range of treatments; getting to meet many different people.

The bad – The days when you are so busy that your legs and feet are aching and there is no time for a break.

Advice for students – Start as a Saturday employee, then after college, get a job in a salon that employs several staff so that you learn from them. Try to stay in your first job for at least a year, which will help you to find out about the industry, how a salon is run, what the job involves, the range of treatments and client types.

a day in the life of...

beauty therapy assistant, Anna

8.30 am Anna arrives at the beauty salon. Her first job is to get all the client lists and record cards ready for each therapist.

9.00 am Reception duty. Anna listens to the answer phone messages, noting them down for the head receptionist to sort out. She welcomes clients and offers them a drink, letting the therapists know that their clients have arrived. She also takes clients through to the treatment rooms if requested by the therapists.

11.00 am Tea break.

11.20 am Anna makes sure all the treatment rooms are well stocked up with tissues, cotton wool squares and towels.

12.00 pm One-hour training session with the head receptionist on booking appointments.

1.00 pm Lunch.

1.45 pm Anna shows clients to the treatment rooms, helps clients with their coats as they leave and gives out salon brochures and price lists. She also tidies the reception area magazines, fills up the coffee machine and replaces brochures when they run out.

3.00 pm Anna sets up for an eyelash perm and then watches it being carried out.

4.00 pm Tea break.

4.20 pm Anna goes out to buy cleaning products and stationery for the salon.

4.45 pm She cleans out the retail display cupboard and re-arranges the display.

5.15 pm She files the day's record cards and tidies the treatment rooms and reception area.

6.00 pm Anna leaves work.

Cruise liner beauty therapist, hair stylist, massage therapist, nail technician

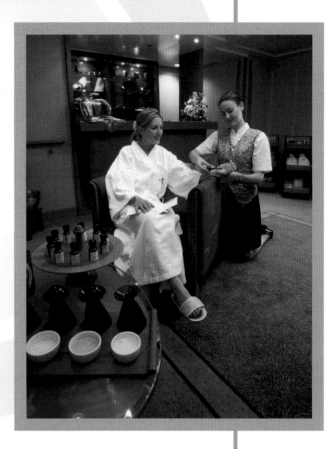

The job – Employment contracts are approximately 8 months' long. Must be physically and emotionally healthy without any romantic ties at home. A medical is required before joining ship.

Training – *Beauty therapists* must offer facial and body massage including electrical face and body treatments; S/NVQ Level 3 required. *Hair stylists* must be qualified to S/NVQ Level 3. *Massage therapists* must offer Swedish Massage with a recognised qualification. *Nail technicians* must offer all nail treatments; either S/NVQ Level 2 or 3 or a recognised nail technician course required.

Pay – Depends on position and experience. Most earnings will come from commission. Passenger tips add to pay.

Hours – Long. Evening work is done on a shift basis.

The good – Excellent career prospects and opportunities for promotion; the chance to travel the world.

promotion: moving up the career ladder to a better job

The bad – Sharing a tiny cabin with another team member for about 8 months. On board ship you are never off duty and the fast-paced life can be hectic and stressful. Homesickness and seasickness are possibilities.

Advice for students – Complete your training, then go into the industry for a couple of years in order to mature and gain experience. During this time try to develop your skills.

a day in the life of...

assistant hairdresser, Carlo

8.30 am Carlo arrives at the salon. His first job is to prepare the perming and tinting products for two clients who are due in at 9 am.

9.00 am He cleans out and disinfects the salon's eight trolleys and changes the sterilising fluid in the jars containing the combs and scissors.

10.30 am Tea break.

10.50 am Carlo shampoos and conditions a client with long hair for the senior stylist Shaz.

11.00 am He assists Shaz by sectioning the long hair and then watches her do the cut.

11.30 am Carlo makes sure the stock cupboard is tidy. He makes a list of stock that he thinks is running out and takes this to the salon manager.

12.00pm Lunch break.

1.00 pm Carlo passes up perm papers and curlers to the stylists, shampoos several clients, places clients under the driers and sweeps the floor.

4.00 pm Reception duty. Carlo shows clients through to the stylists, helps clients with their coats as they leave and gives out salon brochures and price lists.

4.30 pm Danni, another hairdressing assistant, highlights Carlo's hair. Shaz watches and guides them as they are both studying for their S/NVQ Level 2.

6.00 pm Carlo leaves work.

Hair and make-up artist (theatre, media, television/film)

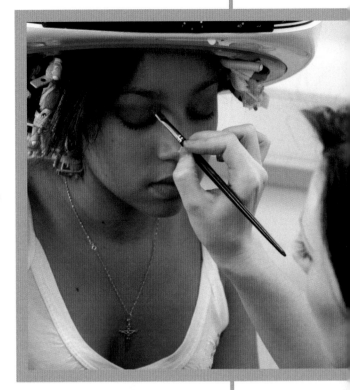

The job – A large part of hair and make-up artistry involves hair as wigs, hairpieces, beards and moustaches. *Theatre work* – applying period and costume make-up for plays and productions and very often detailed fantasy make-up. *Media work* – doing hair and make-up on actors, celebrities, models and presenters; high fashion make-up for magazines, photographic shoots and platform/runway shows. *Television and film work* – designing and making false facial and body features (prosthetics) to change the appearance of an actor, as well as the usual make-up to enhance or alter the actor's look.

Training – Beauty and hairdressing qualifications, followed by a course in TV and film make-up or hairdressing. Become an apprentice to a freelance make-up artist or hairdresser to learn the trade first hand.

Pay – Daily fee, usually starts at £250. Excellent pay for experienced hair and make-up artists.

Hours – Variable, depending on the amount of work on offer.

The good – Possibility of travel to exotic places; meeting famous people; seeing own work on the big screen; seeing own name credited in magazines, shows and television.

The bad – Lots of standing around and waiting, especially in the TV and film industry; pressure to work to strict deadlines; always needing to fit in around other people; some celebrities can be demanding.

Advice for students – You will need a good sense of colour, balance and design. Being creative is essential. Art and History GCSEs and a knowledge of human anatomy would be helpful. Be prepared to work unpaid in amateur dramatics and local theatre companies to gain experience and build up a portfolio to show employers.

TRY IT OUT!

On the following page are some more career opportunities. Research each one and write a job profile like the ones above. Use the same headings:

- The job
- Training
- Pay
- Hours
- The good
- The bad
- Advice for students

Freelance hair stylist or beauty therapist

Some hairdressers and beauty therapists take the salon to the client. This means taking tools and equipment to the client's house or maybe a hospital or care home. People with reduced mobility, such as people with physical disabilities or the elderly, often use the services of freelance hairdressers and beauty therapists.

difficulty with standing and walking

Specialist salons

Some salons concentrate on one or more skill areas, for example a hair salon that specialises in Afro-Caribbean hair or extensions, or a nail bar that specialises in nail techniques.

Health farms, clubs and leisure centres

These concentrate on the health and fitness side of the hair and beauty industry. People usually stay from one night to one week in a health farm in order to get fit and be pampered.

Hotels

Many hotels have hair and beauty salons. Some have their own health spas and leisure clubs. A hotel's main focus is to attract guests by offering a wide range of facilities, including facials and massage treatment and hair services.

Hospitals

Many hospitals have their own hair salon which is open to patients, hospital staff and visitors. Elsewhere, hospitals rely on regular visits to the wards by mobile hairdressers and therapists. Care and rest homes also depend on mobile hair and beauty services.

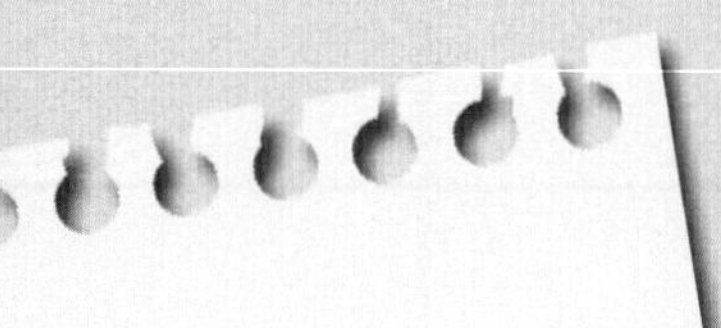

OVER TO YOU...

Write a report about the different jobs in the hair and beauty industry. What jobs are available? Are all of these jobs in salons? Choose **one** job and find out what personal and technical skills are needed to do it. What are the responsibilities?

Education and training

Standards in hairdressing and beauty therapy are set by the Hairdressing and Beauty Industry Authority (Habia). The standards are used as the basis for hair and beauty qualifications, such as S/NVQs. They set out:

- What trainees need to learn.
- What skills trainees need to have.
- What is expected of salon employees.

How and where to train

Whatever job you do, you will need high-quality training on your path to success.

Dear Nat

I'd like to become a beauty therapist or a hairdresser. What qualifications will I need? And how long will it take to qualify?

From Gabriella

Nat says

You'll need to start with the basics. As a 14–16-year-old, this would be S/NVQ Level 1. As a school leaver, you will be able to move on to Level 2 and, finally, to a Level 3 qualification or similar. For Level 1 or 2, it is usually about 1 year. To reach Level 3 standard, it can take up to 3 years. It depends on whether you are studying part time or full time.

Dear Nat

How will I learn and study for my Level 1 Certificate in Salon Services?

From Darren

Nat says

You will study using a variety of methods such as watching demonstrations, practising on each other and clients, assessments, assignments, end of unit tests, coursework and building up a style book.

Once you have achieved your Level 1 Salon Services qualification, there are a number of different ways to train as a hair stylist or beauty therapist.

College of further education

At a further education college, the average length of training on a full-time course is 1 year for S/NVQ Level 2, and 2 years for Level 3. This may depend on:

- Your GCSE grades.
- Any previous experience.
- Your abilities, commitment and attitude.

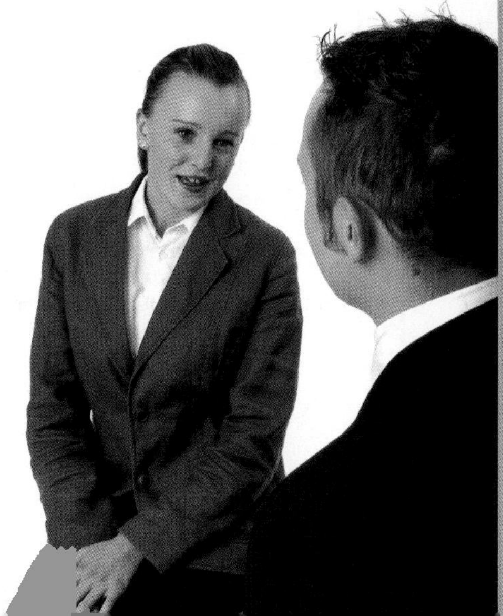

For your college interview make sure you are smart and have a positive attitude

commitment: how prepared you are to do something

attitude: how much you want to do something

working at a fast pace

Private training centre

Private training centre courses are usually shorter and more intensive with smaller class sizes. Not all private centres offer nationally recognised qualifications, so you should check what qualification you will get at the end of the course.

TOP TIP

There are a wide range of courses and qualifications in the UK. It depends on which type of training is best for you. If you don't like exams but prefer to be assessed regularly on your work, then an S/NVQ might be your best choice. If you prefer to sit final examinations, then there are courses that offer this.

Apprenticeships in hair and beauty

These are aimed at 16–24-year-olds. The training is work-based, so it provides an excellent opportunity for work experience as well as study. The trainee usually attends college one day per week and is in paid employment for the rest of the week.

To find out more, contact your local Learning and Skills Council (LSC) or careers office. Look out for employers and training organisations advertising for apprenticeships. For a link to the LSC's apprentices' website, visit www.heinemann.co.uk/hotlinks and enter the express code 3071P.

Dear Nat

What can I do when I have got my Level 1 in Salon Services?

From Emily

Nat says

You can work as an assistant to a hairdresser or beauty therapist but it is worth going on with your studies to become a fully qualified hair stylist or therapist. You have lots of opportunities for different careers, and the more you study, the more choices you will have. S/NVQs are good as they allow you to build up your skills in steps.

Hair and beauty qualifications

S/NVQs

When you read the job profiles earlier in the unit, you probably noticed that to do most of the jobs you would need to have a beauty therapy or hairdressing NVQ – national vocational qualification (SVQ in Scotland), or similar. Vocational qualifications are 'what you can do' qualifications. That means they tell the employer the skills and knowledge you have and that you can do a particular kind of work to a certain standard. S/NVQs are divided into different levels. The training and career pathways show the level you would need to do different jobs in hairdressing and beauty therapy.

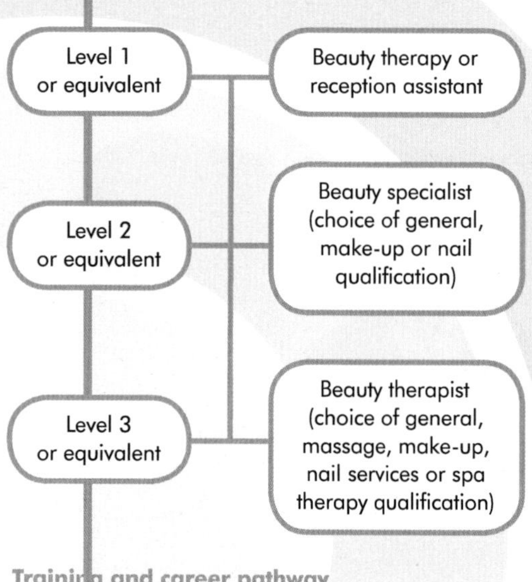

Training and career pathway for beauty therapy

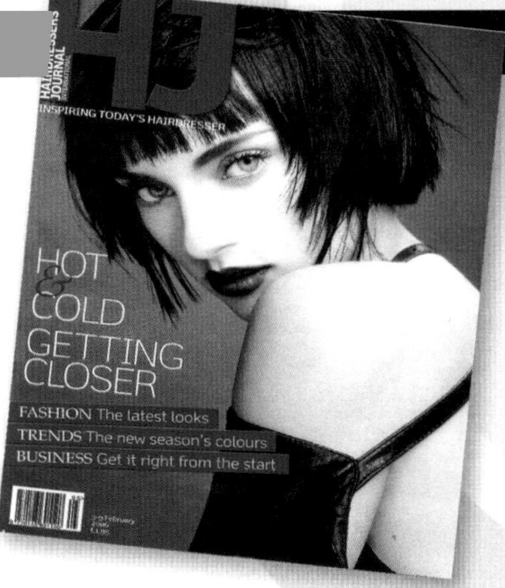

A hairdressing trade journal

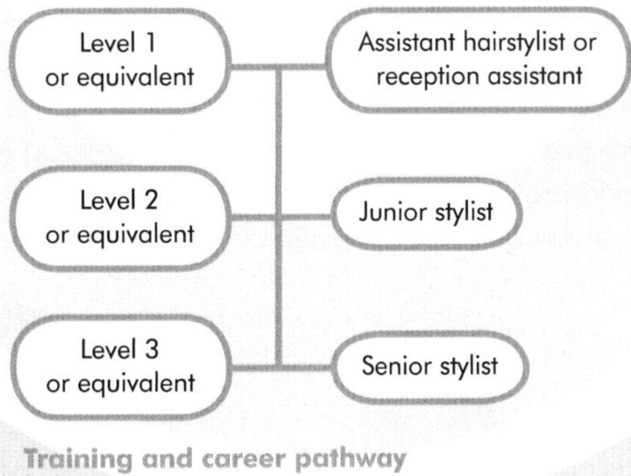

Training and career pathway for hairdressing

Developing your career

Once you have got your Level 1 Certificate in Salon Services, you will need to think carefully about where you want to go next. You will probably move on to S/NVQ Level 1 or 2 or a similar qualification. Whatever you choose to do, remember that up-to-date knowledge and skills are very important in this fast-changing industry. Once qualified, you must be prepared to regularly re-train and learn new skills, or you will be left behind. In order to make choices about your career you will need to have good quality information about careers, education and training.

OVER TO YOU...

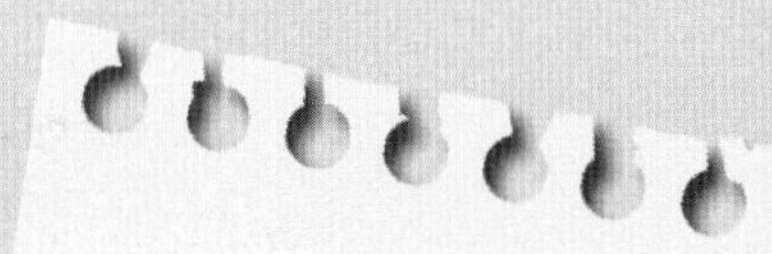

Find out what the staffing structure is like in a typical salon. How do different jobs link together? Who does each person report to? Where would you fit in? As your skills and responsibilities increase, what options might be open to you? What training or qualifications might you need? Write a report on what you have found.

Trade journals

Trade journals (example shown above) are written for everyone involved in the hair and beauty industry and are a great way to get good quality information. The journals will keep you up-to-date with the latest treatments, hair and beauty products, make-up and hair trends, events and personalities in the trade. It will help you to become a regular reader of some of the journals below:

Health and Beauty
Professional Beauty
Warpaint
Professional Nails
Hairdressers Journal International
Vitality (available to members of British Association of Beauty Therapy and Cosmetology (BABTAC))
Scratch
Salon Today
Guild News

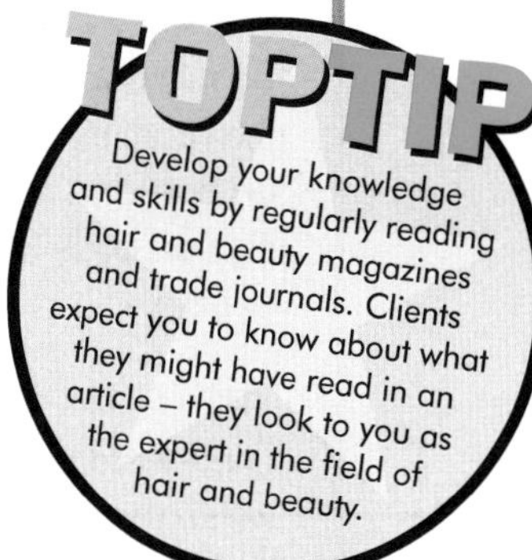

TOPTIP
Develop your knowledge and skills by regularly reading hair and beauty magazines and trade journals. Clients expect you to know about what they might have read in an article – they look to you as the expert in the field of hair and beauty.

Connexions

Connexions offers careers, work and job advice and information to 13–19-year-olds living in England. It also provides support up to the age of 25 for people who have learning difficulties or disabilities (or both). Advisers visit schools throughout the country to give confidential support and guidance in career decisions, personal problems and financial guidance. To find out more, visit the Connexions website – for a link to this website go to www.heinemann.co.uk/hotlinks and enter the express code 3071P.

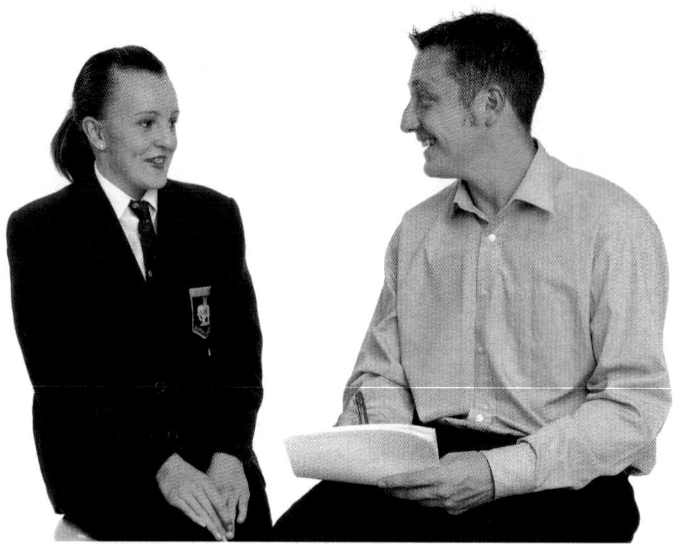

A Connexions adviser chats to a student

Hairdressing and Beauty Industry Authority (Habia)

Habia provides guidance on careers, business development, legislation, salon safety and equal opportunities. Contact Habia at the address below to obtain leaflets on qualifications and careers available.

Habia, Oxford House, Sixth Avenue, Sky Business Park, Robin Hood Airport, Doncaster DN9 3GG. Tel: 08452 306080

For a link to the Habia website, visit www.heinemann.co.uk/hotlinks and enter the express code 3071P.

Exhibitions and competitions

To find out more about the very latest trends and products in the hair and beauty industry, try to visit some of the major hair and beauty exhibitions such as Professional Beauty and Salon International. For a link to the news and information website for the main exhibitions in the hair and beauty industry and a website giving information on past and future exhibitions, visit www.heinemann.co.uk/hotlinks and enter the express code 3071P. Hair and beauty competitions are also a good way to keep up to date.

The Awarding Bodies

The Awarding Bodies are organisations that provide recognised qualifications within the hair and beauty industry. To obtain leaflets giving information about the qualifications they offer, contact each of the Awarding Bodies listed below.

To link to their websites, visit www.heinemann.co.uk/hotlinks and enter the express code 3071P

VTCT (Vocational Training and Charitable Trust), Unit 11, Brickfield Trading Estate, Brickfield Lane, Chandlers Ford, Hampshire SO53 4DR. 023 8027 1733.

City & Guilds, 1 Giltspur Street, London EC1A 9DD. Tel: 020 7294 2800

International Therapy Examination Council (ITEC), 4 Heathfield Terrace, Chiswick, London W4 4JE. Tel: 020 8994 4141

Confederation of International Beauty Therapy and Cosmetology (CIBTAC), Meteor Court, Barnett Way, Gloucester GL4 3GG. Tel: 01452 623114

Comite International d'Esthetique et de Cosmetologie (CIDESCO), The Secretariat, Witikonerstrasse 365, 8053 Zurich, Switzerland. Tel: +41 44 380 00 75

Edexcel, Stewart House, 32 Russell Square, London WC1B 5DN. Tel: 0870 240 9800

OVER TO YOU...

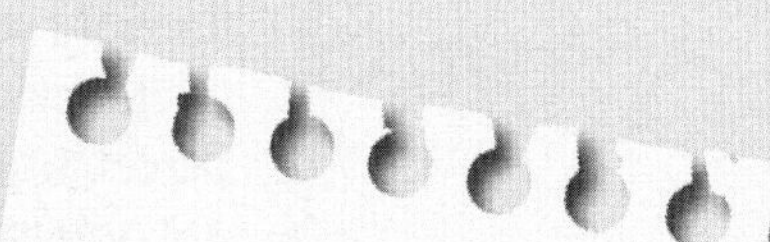

Write a report about the main organisations that provide information on working in the hair and beauty industry. Who is the main representative? Are there any professional and awarding bodies in hair and beauty? If you can, collect publicity about the organisations for your report. Don't forget to refer to Connexions and the services they offer.

Employee rights

Pay and perks

National minimum wage

Since 1999, by law, employers must not pay employees less than the national minimum wage. From 1 October 2005, the national minimum wage for employees aged 18–21 years in recognised training was at least £4.25 per hour and for employees aged 22 years and over, at least £5.05 per hour. For employees aged 22 and over and in recognised training, employers only have to pay £4.25 per hour for the first 6 months, then the national minimum wage. If you are aged 16 or 17 you will be entitled to at least £3 per hour, but if you are on an Apprenticeship Scheme, you will not be entitled to the minimum wage until you are 19 years old.

For more information visit the Department of Trade and Industry (DTI) and Connexions websites. For a link to both these websites, visit www.heinemann.co.uk/hotlinks and enter the express code 3071P.

Your pay

At the time of writing (November 2005), a newly qualified beauty therapist or hairdresser could earn about £9,000 per year and experienced therapists between £12,000 and £18,000 a year.

These figures are only a guideline and much higher salaries are now being earned in an industry that was once very poorly paid. Jobs such as product trainers and spa managers can demand excellent wages in line with their experience and expertise.

Perks

A job in the hair and beauty industry has always provided a bonus – the chance to be pampered yourself! Although this is a perk of the job, it is important that you look well-groomed at all times. If there is a gap in the appointments column and all other jobs are done, then it is accepted that staff can carry out treatments or practise new skills on each other as long as it does not affect their work.

not part of your wages

Staff treatments should never be put in the appointment column if a paying client could fill the space. Each company will have its own rules on staff treatments. It may be that employees are asked to make a small payment towards the products used in the treatment.

Some companies offer incentives on top of wages, such as paying commission to staff on every product they sell. Other companies reward employees who make the business a lot of money through treatments and sales by paying them a percentage of the business's takings. This not only boosts employees' wages but also helps the salon to keep its best staff.

things to encourage staff to work harder

extra money on top of wages for products sold or treatments

Further perks are tips, which are very common in hair and beauty salons. These are small sums of money paid directly to staff by clients when they are pleased with their treatment. They are in addition to the cost of the service or treatment.

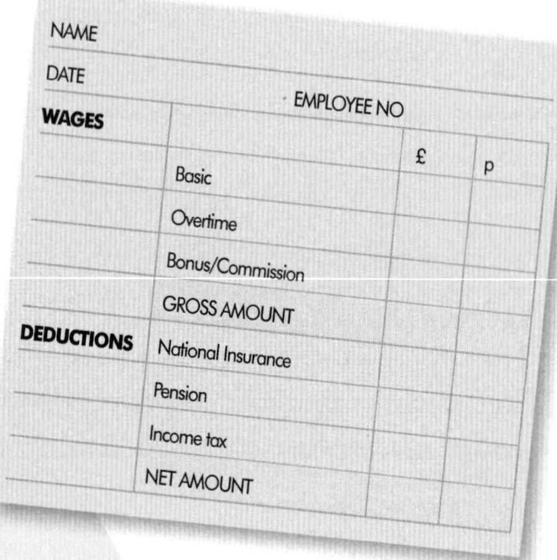

NAME			
DATE	EMPLOYEE NO		
WAGES		£	p
	Basic		
	Overtime		
	Bonus/Commission		
	GROSS AMOUNT		
DEDUCTIONS	National Insurance		
	Pension		
	Income tax		
	NET AMOUNT		

A typical pay slip

Your rights

As an employee, you have rights at work, which protect you from unfair pay and conditions. You also have the right to be treated fairly and to work in a safe environment.

place

These are the main employee rights:

- The right to receive the national minimum wage.
- The right to have a contract of employment.
- The right not to be dismissed unfairly.
- The right to be given a written reason if dismissed.
- Maternity rights – includes time off work before and after the birth.
- The right not to be discriminated against because of ethnic origin, sex, religion, disability, hours worked or pay.
- The right to equal pay.
- The right to join a trade union.
- The right of confidentiality. Personal work records may only be seen by the person who is responsible for staff information within the business.

to treat someone differently or unfairly

race, nationality or culture

privacy

Employees also have a duty not to discriminate against others, cause risks to health and safety or break confidentiality about the business.

Changes in an employee's personal life

Employees must tell employers about:

- Changes to their health and well-being.
- Changes to their address and contact details.
- If they have been in trouble with the law.

An employee has a duty to tell his or her employer about these changes because they could affect the type of work that can be done, the hours and the ability to contact the employee.

Confidentiality

Staff learn a lot about a business when they work there. They need information about the business in order to do their job, and they will have access to confidential information during their employment. It is very important that employees are trustworthy and loyal.

Types of confidential information that an employee might see or learn about include:

- Customer information, e.g. names of clients, their addresses and contact details. Treatments or services they have received, payment history and/or money owed.
- Financial information, e.g. daily/weekly takings.
- Current or future plans, e.g. special selling methods, new products or services.
- Management problems.
- Information about business partners.

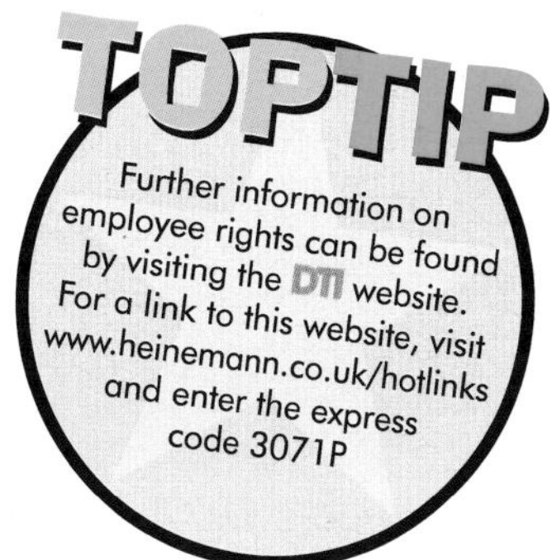

TOPTIP
Further information on employee rights can be found by visiting the DTI website. For a link to this website, visit www.heinemann.co.uk/hotlinks and enter the express code 3071P

Department of Trade and Industry

Contract of employment

When you accept a job, the company must give you a written contract of employment. By law, your employer must give you this within 2 months of starting work.

The contract will include:

- Names and addresses of the employer and employee.
- Date the job started.
- Job title and description, covering specific responsibilities.
- Hours of work.
- Length and type of employment, e.g. temporary maternity cover for 6 months, permanent contract.
- Place or places of work.
- Salary.
- Holiday entitlement.
- Method of pay, e.g. monthly direct into your bank, weekly wage.
- Sickness and injury pay.
- Length of notice required (may be anything from 2 weeks to 3 months depending on the company).
- Details of any pension schemes.
- Disciplinary or grievance procedures.

rights

privacy

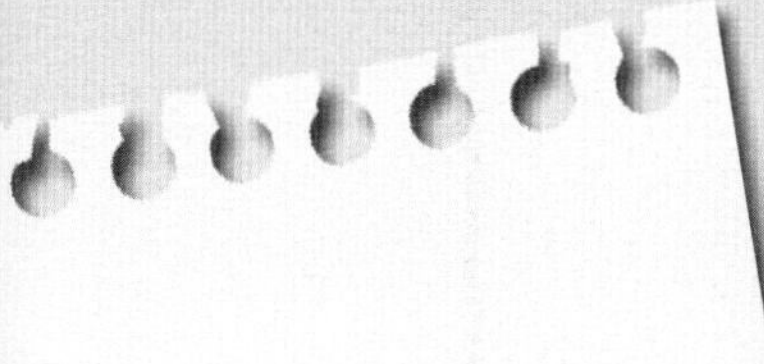

OVER TO YOU...

Write a short report about your rights and responsibilities as an employee. You should also include information about the contents of a typical contract, minimum wage and working time regulations. Do you think working in a salon might affect your rights and responsibilities?

Check what you know...

Watch out! Some questions have more than one correct answer.

1. Habia stands for:
   - [ ] Hairdressing and Barbering Industry Association
   - [ ] Health and Beauty Industry Association
   - [ ] Hairdressing and Beauty Industry Authority
2. What is information about a job called?
   - [ ] contract of employment
   - [ ] condition of particulars
   - [ ] confidentiality contract
3. What information should be on a pay slip?
   - [ ] name, age and hours you worked
   - [ ] amount you earned, any commission and deductions
   - [ ] amount you earned and lost
4. What is the national minimum wage for 16 and 17 year olds?
   - [ ] £5.10 [ ] £4.10 [ ] £3.00
5. What does NVQ stand for?
   - [ ] national verifying qualification
   - [ ] never very quick
   - [ ] national vocational qualification
6. Why is it important to keep studying once you have qualified?
   - [ ] to keep up to date with new treatments, products and information
   - [ ] because your qualification will get out of date
   - [ ] because there are better people at the job
7. If you have a Level 1 qualification you could work as a:
   - [ ] beauty therapist or hairdresser
   - [ ] a salon assisstant
   - [ ] a barber
8. If you need help or support with your studying or learning, you can get advice from:
   - [ ] a Habia advisor
   - [ ] a doctor
   - [ ] a Connexions advisor
9. Confidential information is:
   - [ ] private information
   - [ ] important information
   - [ ] secret information
10. A perk of the job is:
    - [ ] being able to leave early when your boss isn't there
    - [ ] having treatments done on yourself when it's quiet
    - [ ] taking things from the stock cupboard to use at home